Hormonal Harmony Manual

A Comprehensive Guide to Promoting Healthy Hormones for Women Over 40

By

Calvin M. Duncan

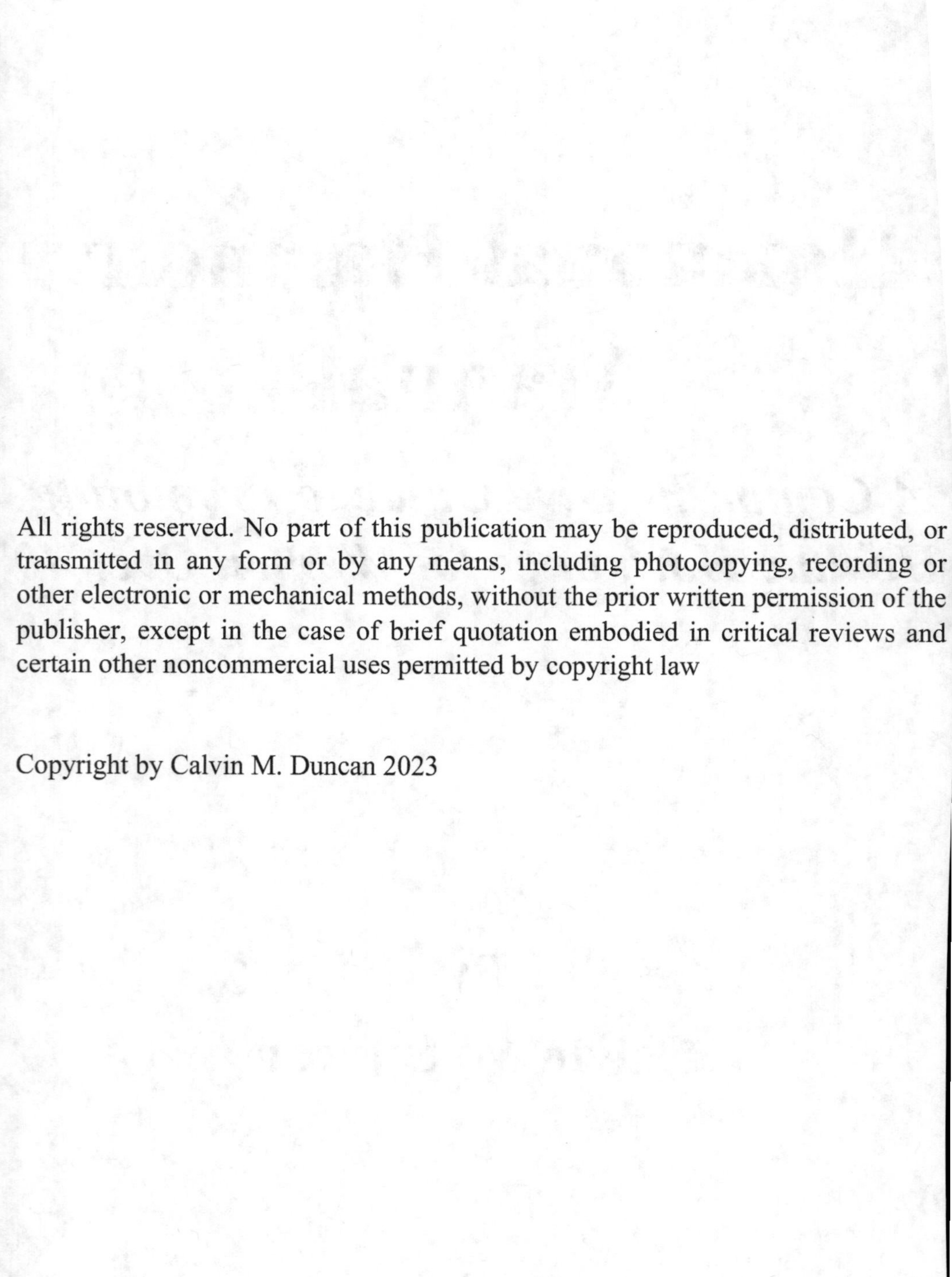

Table of Contents

INTRODUCTION

In the intricate tapestry of a woman's life, the chapter that unfolds around the age of 40 is often marked by profound changes—physiological, emotional, and psychological. This pivotal period, often referred to as the "over-40" phase, brings with it a unique set of challenges and transformations, chief among them being the intricate dance of hormonal fluctuations. It is during this juncture that the Hormonal Harmony Manual emerges as a guiding light, a comprehensive guide meticulously crafted to empower women with the knowledge and strategies needed to navigate the intricate landscape of hormonal changes and foster a state of well-being.

The journey into the world of hormones is a journey into the very essence of a woman's biology. Hormones, the chemical messengers coursing through the bloodstream, orchestrate a symphony of physiological processes, influencing everything from mood and metabolism to reproductive health and bone density. Understanding the profound impact of hormonal changes on women's health is the first step toward unlocking the secrets to a harmonious and fulfilling life beyond 40.

As we embark on this exploration, it is essential to recognize the uniqueness of each woman's hormonal journey. No two experiences are identical, and the Hormonal Harmony Manual seeks to embrace this diversity, offering insights and strategies that can be tailored to individual needs. Whether one is approaching perimenopause, navigating the challenges of menopause, or simply seeking to optimize hormonal health in the years beyond 40, this handbook serves as a companion, providing knowledge, support, and actionable steps.

Why, one might ask, is hormonal health of particular significance for women over 40? The answer lies in the pivotal role hormones play in orchestrating various physiological functions. Hormones act as messengers, transmitting signals between different organs and tissues, regulating processes such as metabolism, immune function, and the menstrual cycle. Understanding the delicate balance required for optimal hormonal health is akin to deciphering the language of the body.

The over-40 phase is often associated with significant hormonal transitions, particularly in the realms of perimenopause and menopause. These transitions bring about a decline in the production of key hormones such as estrogen and progesterone, leading to a host of physical and emotional changes. The repercussions of these changes extend beyond the reproductive system, influencing bone health, cardiovascular function, and mental well-being.

It is crucial to recognize that the hormonal journey is not a linear path but a dynamic and individualized process. Some women may breeze through these changes with minimal disruption, while others may face more pronounced challenges. The Hormonal Harmony Manual acknowledges the diversity of these experiences, aiming to empower women with the tools to navigate their unique hormonal landscapes.

Knowledge is a powerful tool, and the Hormonal Harmony Manual is founded on the belief that empowering women with information about their bodies fosters a sense of agency and control. This handbook serves as a comprehensive resource, offering evidence-based insights into the mechanisms of hormonal changes, their impact on health, and strategies to promote harmony.

In an era where information is abundant but not always easily accessible, the Handbook distills complex scientific concepts into digestible and practical information. It bridges the gap between the latest research findings and their real-world application, ensuring that women can make informed decisions about their health. By understanding the intricacies of hormonal changes, women are better equipped to engage in meaningful conversations with healthcare professionals, ask pertinent questions, and actively participate in decisions about their well-being.

The Hormonal Harmony Manual is organized with a holistic approach, recognizing that hormonal health is a multifaceted tapestry woven from various threads—nutrition, lifestyle, mental well-being, and medical interventions. Each chapter is designed to unravel a different aspect of this tapestry, providing a comprehensive understanding of the factors influencing hormonal health.

The journey begins with an exploration of Hormone Basics, laying the foundation by introducing key hormones and their roles in the body. It then navigates through the Signs of Hormonal Imbalance, offering insights into recognizing and interpreting the signals that the body may send during periods of hormonal fluctuation.

Moving forward, the Handbook delves into Hormone Repair Strategies, exploring the crucial role of nutrition, lifestyle modifications, and exercise in promoting hormonal balance. It provides practical tips and actionable steps that women can incorporate into their daily lives to support their hormonal well-being.

A significant section is devoted to Hormone-Friendly Recipes, recognizing the intimate connection between what we eat and our hormonal health. The Handbook offers nutritious meal plans and delicious recipes designed to nourish the body and support hormonal balance.

Natural Supplements and Therapies constitute another dimension of the Handbook, shedding light on alternative approaches to hormonal health. From herbal remedies to holistic therapies, this section provides insights into complementary methods that women may consider on their journey.

Hormone Testing and Monitoring are explored in detail, emphasizing the importance of regular check-ups and understanding test results. This section empowers women to take an active role in monitoring their hormonal health and seeking timely interventions when needed.

Personalized Hormone Care Plans take center stage as the Handbook guides women in tailoring strategies to their individual needs. Recognizing that there is no one-size-fits-all solution, this section encourages a personalized and sustainable approach to hormonal well-being.

Real-Life Success Stories add a human touch to the Handbook, featuring narratives of women who have navigated their hormonal journeys successfully. These stories inspire and provide practical insights into the challenges and triumphs of real women.

The Handbook concludes with Frequently Asked Questions, addressing common concerns and providing expert insights. It also offers a curated list of Resources and Further Reading, guiding women to explore additional information and connect with supportive communities.

In essence, the Hormonal Harmony Manual is more than a compilation of information; it is a companion on the journey to hormonal well-being. It is a roadmap that empowers women to traverse the diverse landscapes of hormonal changes with resilience, knowledge, and a sense of purpose.

As we embark on this exploration of hormonal health for women over 40, it is essential to recognize that this journey is not a solitary one. The Hormonal Harmony Manual is an invitation to join a community of women who share similar experiences, concerns, and aspirations. It is a testament to the resilience of the female body and spirit, acknowledging that every woman has the capacity to navigate the intricacies of hormonal changes and emerge stronger and more empowered.

May the pages of the Hormonal Harmony Manual serve as a source of inspiration, knowledge, and practical guidance. May it empower women to embrace their bodies, celebrate the wisdom that comes with age, and embark on a journey of holistic well-being. Together, let us navigate the pathways of hormonal harmony, fostering a future where women over 40 not only thrive but flourish in the fullness of their health and vitality.

CHAPTER ONE

Understanding Hormonal Changes

Hormones play a pivotal role in the intricate symphony of the human body, orchestrating a myriad of physiological processes that influence our health and well-being. As individuals approach and navigate their way through the age of 40 and beyond, hormonal changes become a significant aspect of their biological journey. In this exploration, we will delve into the complexities of hormonal fluctuations, examining the mechanisms behind these changes and the profound impact they can have on both physical and mental aspects of life.

The Endocrine System: A Symphony of Signals

At the core of hormonal changes lies the endocrine system, a network of glands that produce and release hormones into the bloodstream. These chemical messengers travel throughout the body, binding to specific receptors and influencing the function of various organs and tissues. The endocrine system includes glands such as the pituitary, thyroid, adrenal, and reproductive glands, each playing a unique role in maintaining homeostasis.

Puberty and Reproductive Years: The Prelude

The journey of hormonal changes begins in adolescence with the onset of puberty. This transformative phase is marked by the awakening of the reproductive system, orchestrated by the release of hormones such as estrogen and testosterone. Puberty not only leads to physical changes like the development of secondary sexual characteristics but also sets the stage for the reproductive years.

During the reproductive years, the menstrual cycle becomes a central hormonal event for women. The interplay between follicle-stimulating hormone (FSH), luteinizing hormone (LH), estrogen, and progesterone regulates the menstrual cycle, preparing the body for potential pregnancy. This cyclical process is a delicate dance of hormonal coordination, with each phase serving a specific purpose in the intricate reproductive symphony.

Perimenopause: The Prelude to Change

As women approach their 40s, they enter a transitional phase known as perimenopause. This period, typically lasting several years before menopause, is characterized by erratic hormonal fluctuations. The ovaries gradually reduce their production of estrogen and progesterone, leading

to irregular menstrual cycles and a variety of symptoms such as hot flashes, mood swings, and changes in libido.

Perimenopause is a time of adaptation, and the body strives to find a new hormonal equilibrium. While some women may experience mild symptoms, others may face more pronounced challenges. The variability in individual experiences during perimenopause underscores the importance of understanding hormonal changes on a personalized level.

Menopause: Navigating New Horizons

Menopause marks the cessation of menstruation and the end of the reproductive years. The average age of menopause is around 51, but it can occur earlier or later for some women. During menopause, the ovaries cease to release eggs, and hormonal levels, particularly estrogen and progesterone, decline significantly.

The absence of these hormones triggers a cascade of changes in the body, leading to a range of symptoms. Common manifestations include vaginal dryness, sleep disturbances, mood changes, and an increased risk of conditions like osteoporosis and cardiovascular disease. Understanding the dynamics of hormonal changes during menopause is crucial for women as they navigate this transformative phase of life.

Hormonal Impact on Physical Health

Hormonal changes extend their influence beyond the reproductive system, affecting various aspects of physical health. The decline in estrogen during menopause, for instance, is associated with changes in bone density, potentially leading to osteoporosis. Hormones also play a role in regulating metabolism, and imbalances can contribute to weight gain and alterations in body composition.

Moreover, hormonal fluctuations can impact the cardiovascular system. Estrogen, in particular, has cardioprotective effects, and its decline during menopause may contribute to an increased risk of heart disease. Understanding these connections is essential for implementing strategies to support overall physical well-being during and after periods of hormonal transition.

Hormonal Impact on Mental Health

The intricate interplay between hormones and mental health is a topic of increasing interest and research. Hormonal changes can influence mood, cognition, and emotional well-being. For example, fluctuations in estrogen levels have been linked to an increased susceptibility to mood disorders such as depression and anxiety.

The menopausal transition, characterized by hormonal upheavals, is a period when many women report changes in mood and emotional resilience. Sleep disturbances, which are common during hormonal changes, can further contribute to emotional challenges. By understanding the connection between hormones and mental health, individuals can explore holistic approaches to support their emotional well-being during times of hormonal flux.

Managing Hormonal Changes: A Holistic Approach

Effectively managing hormonal changes involves a holistic approach that addresses both the physical and emotional aspects of well-being. Nutrition plays a crucial role, and adopting a balanced diet rich in nutrients can support hormonal balance. Nutrients such as omega-3 fatty acids, vitamin D, and antioxidants contribute to overall hormonal health and can be obtained through a diverse and wholesome diet.

Lifestyle modifications also play a significant role in navigating hormonal changes. Regular physical activity has been shown to have positive effects on hormonal balance, reducing symptoms like hot flashes and contributing to overall mental well-being. Adequate sleep is another crucial component, as it allows the body to regulate hormonal release and supports the restoration of physiological balance.

In addition to lifestyle changes, some women may explore hormonal therapies or natural supplements to manage symptoms. Hormone replacement therapy (HRT), for example, involves the administration of hormones like estrogen and progesterone to alleviate menopausal symptoms. However, the decision to pursue such interventions should be individualized, considering factors like overall health and potential risks.

Empowering Women Through Knowledge

Understanding hormonal changes is empowering, providing individuals with the knowledge to navigate the various stages of life with resilience and informed decision-making. As research continues to unveil the intricate connections between hormones and health, a comprehensive understanding of hormonal changes becomes increasingly vital.

Educational initiatives and open conversations about hormonal health can contribute to a supportive environment where individuals feel empowered to seek information, share experiences, and make choices that align with their well-being. By embracing the nuances of hormonal changes, women can embark on a journey of self-discovery and well-being, fostering a sense of control and confidence in the face of transformative biological shifts.

Importance of Healthy Hormones After 40

The age of 40 serves as a significant milestone in a woman's life, signaling a period of transition and change. It marks the intersection of experience and a subtle turning point in health and well-being. One of the key aspects that come into focus during this phase is the delicate balance of hormones within the female body. The importance of healthy hormones after 40 cannot be overstated, as these chemical messengers play a pivotal role in orchestrating various physiological functions that contribute to overall vitality, emotional well-being, and longevity.

Before delving into the importance of healthy hormones after 40, it is crucial to comprehend the nature of hormonal changes that occur during this stage of life. The endocrine system, a complex network of glands that produce and release hormones, undergoes subtle but impactful shifts as women approach and navigate their way through their 40s and beyond.

The journey typically begins with perimenopause, a transitional phase that precedes menopause. Perimenopause is characterized by fluctuations in hormone levels, particularly estrogen and progesterone, leading to irregular menstrual cycles and a range of symptoms such as hot flashes, mood swings, and changes in libido. Menopause, the cessation of menstruation, follows, and with it comes a significant decline in the production of these key hormones.

These hormonal changes, while a natural and inevitable part of the aging process, bring about a cascade of effects throughout the body. The implications extend beyond the reproductive system, influencing bone health, cardiovascular function, metabolism, and mental well-being. As such, maintaining healthy hormones after 40 becomes a cornerstone of promoting overall health and quality of life.

Bone Health and Hormones

One of the critical areas where hormonal changes after 40 have a pronounced impact is bone health. Estrogen, a hormone primarily produced by the ovaries, plays a crucial role in maintaining bone density. As estrogen levels decline during perimenopause and menopause, the rate of bone loss accelerates, leading to an increased risk of osteoporosis.

Osteoporosis is a condition characterized by weakened and porous bones, making them more susceptible to fractures. The decline in bone density can be particularly concerning for women as they age, as fractures and bone-related issues can significantly affect mobility and overall quality

of life. Maintaining healthy hormones, therefore, becomes a key strategy in preserving bone health and preventing the onset of osteoporosis.

Cardiovascular Health and Hormones

Hormones also exert a profound influence on cardiovascular health, and the changes that occur after 40 can impact the risk of heart disease. Estrogen, in particular, has cardioprotective effects, contributing to the dilation of blood vessels and the maintenance of healthy cholesterol levels. As estrogen levels decline during menopause, women become more susceptible to cardiovascular issues.

Postmenopausal women face an increased risk of conditions such as hypertension, elevated cholesterol levels, and atherosclerosis. The interconnected relationship between hormones and cardiovascular health underscores the importance of proactive measures to support hormonal balance and reduce the risk of heart disease. Healthy lifestyle choices, including regular exercise, a balanced diet, and stress management, play a crucial role in promoting cardiovascular well-being after 40.

Metabolism and Weight Management

Hormones play a central role in regulating metabolism, the process by which the body converts food into energy. Changes in hormonal balance, particularly the decline in estrogen, can impact metabolism and contribute to weight gain, especially around the abdominal area. This shift in fat distribution is not only a cosmetic concern but also a potential risk factor for metabolic disorders such as insulin resistance and type 2 diabetes.

Maintaining a healthy weight through a combination of regular physical activity and a balanced diet is essential for overall well-being after 40. Hormonal changes can make weight management more challenging, but adopting a proactive and sustainable approach can mitigate these challenges and support metabolic health.

Mental Well-being and Hormones

The intricate interplay between hormones and mental health is a dynamic aspect of the hormonal changes that occur after 40. Estrogen, in particular, has been linked to neurotransmitters that influence mood, cognition, and emotional well-being. The decline in estrogen levels during perimenopause and menopause can contribute to symptoms such as mood swings, irritability, and an increased risk of mood disorders such as depression and anxiety.

Cognitive functions, including memory and concentration, may also be affected by hormonal changes. The importance of maintaining healthy hormones goes beyond physical health and extends to preserving cognitive function and emotional resilience. Strategies such as regular

exercise, adequate sleep, and stress management play a crucial role in supporting mental well-being during hormonal transitions.

Reproductive and Sexual Health

While the cessation of menstruation is a natural part of the aging process, the impact of hormonal changes on reproductive and sexual health should not be overlooked. Hormones play a central role in the health of the reproductive organs, and their decline can lead to changes in vaginal health, including dryness and thinning of the vaginal walls.

Maintaining healthy hormones after 40 is essential for supporting reproductive and sexual well-being. Open communication with healthcare professionals can help address concerns and explore options for managing symptoms. Additionally, embracing a positive attitude toward changes in sexual health and seeking support when needed contribute to a fulfilling and satisfying post-reproductive life.

Strategies for Supporting Healthy Hormones After 40

Given the multifaceted impact of hormonal changes on various aspects of health, adopting proactive strategies to support hormonal balance becomes imperative after 40. These strategies encompass lifestyle choices, dietary considerations, and, in some cases, medical interventions. Here are key approaches to promote healthy hormones:

1. Nutrient-Rich Diet: A balanced and nutrient-rich diet plays a fundamental role in supporting hormonal health. Essential nutrients such as omega-3 fatty acids, vitamins, and minerals contribute to the production and regulation of hormones. Emphasizing a variety of fruits, vegetables, whole grains, and lean proteins provides the body with the building blocks for optimal hormonal function.

2. Regular Physical Activity: Exercise is a powerful modulator of hormonal balance. Regular physical activity not only supports metabolic health but also promotes the release of endorphins, the body's natural mood enhancers. Both aerobic exercises and strength training contribute to overall well-being and hormonal harmony.

3. Stress Management: Chronic stress can disrupt hormonal balance, leading to a cascade of physiological effects. Implementing stress-management techniques such as meditation, deep breathing exercises, and mindfulness can help mitigate the impact of stress on hormones.

4. Adequate Sleep: Quality sleep is essential for hormonal regulation and overall health. Hormones involved in the sleep-wake cycle, such as melatonin, play a crucial role in maintaining circadian rhythms. Establishing a consistent sleep routine and creating a conducive sleep environment contribute to hormonal balance.

5. Hormone Replacement Therapy (HRT): In some cases, healthcare professionals may recommend hormone replacement therapy to address specific symptoms associated with hormonal

decline. HRT involves the administration of hormones such as estrogen and progesterone to alleviate symptoms like hot flashes, mood swings, and vaginal dryness. The decision to pursue HRT should be individualized and made in consultation with a healthcare provider, considering factors such as overall health and potential risks.

6. Complementary Therapies: Some women explore complementary therapies such as herbal supplements, acupuncture, or biofeedback to support hormonal balance. While research on the effectiveness of these approaches varies, some women find relief from symptoms through these alternative methods. It is essential to consult with healthcare professionals before incorporating complementary therapies into a wellness plan.

7. Regular Health Check-ups: Monitoring hormonal health through regular check-ups and screenings is crucial for early detection and intervention. Regular gynecological examinations, bone density tests, and cardiovascular assessments contribute to a proactive approach to health maintenance.

The Holistic Approach to Healthy Hormones

Recognizing the interconnectedness of various aspects of health, a holistic approach is paramount when aiming to maintain healthy hormones after 40. Rather than isolating hormonal health from other facets of well-being, this approach acknowledges that lifestyle choices, mental well-being, and medical interventions all play integral roles in supporting hormonal balance.

Holistic health promotes an understanding that the body operates as a unified system, with each element influencing the others. Adopting a balanced lifestyle that includes regular exercise, a nutritious diet, stress management, and adequate sleep creates a foundation for hormonal harmony. In this context, the importance of a positive mindset and self-care practices cannot be overstated, as they contribute to emotional resilience and overall well-being.

The Journey of Empowerment

The transition beyond 40 is not merely a journey of aging but a journey of empowerment. Recognizing the importance of healthy hormones during this phase is an acknowledgment of the body's wisdom and resilience. It is an invitation to embrace the changes that come with age, armed with knowledge and proactive strategies to support well-being.

Empowerment comes from understanding that hormonal changes are a natural part of life, and each woman's journey is unique. By fostering a sense of agency and actively participating in decisions related to health, women can navigate the transitions of perimenopause and menopause with grace and confidence.

As women embrace the significance of healthy hormones after 40, they contribute not only to their individual well-being but also to a broader societal shift. Open conversations, awareness, and

support networks create an environment where women feel empowered to prioritize their health and share their experiences. In doing so, they become advocates for hormonal health, challenging societal norms and contributing to a narrative that celebrates the diverse and transformative journeys of women over 40.

In Conclusion

The importance of healthy hormones after 40 cannot be overstated, as these chemical messengers play a pivotal role in shaping the physical, emotional, and mental well-being of women. The transitions of perimenopause and menopause bring about changes that ripple through various aspects of health, highlighting the interconnectedness of the body's systems.

Maintaining healthy hormones is not about thwarting the aging process but about navigating it with resilience, knowledge, and a commitment to well-being. It involves embracing a holistic approach that addresses lifestyle, nutrition, mental well-being, and, when necessary, medical interventions. By doing so, women can empower themselves to not only weather the hormonal changes that come with age but to thrive and embrace the fullness of life beyond 40.

As the journey unfolds, it is a testament to the strength and wisdom inherent in every woman. Through understanding, empowerment, and proactive choices, women can navigate the terrain of hormonal changes with grace, vitality, and an unwavering commitment to their own flourishing. The importance of healthy hormones after 40, therefore, becomes a rallying cry for a new narrative—one that celebrates the resilience, beauty, and strength of women in the prime of their lives.

CHAPTER TWO

Overview of Key Hormones in Women

The human body is a marvel of biological complexity, with an intricate system of chemical messengers known as hormones orchestrating various physiological functions. In the context of women's health, understanding the roles and interactions of key hormones is essential, as these molecules play a pivotal role in regulating reproductive processes, supporting overall well-being, and influencing various aspects of daily life.

Estrogen: The Feminine Essence

Estrogen, often considered the quintessential female hormone, plays a central role in the development and regulation of the female reproductive system. Produced primarily by the ovaries, estrogen exists in different forms—estradiol, estrone, and estriol. Across the menstrual cycle, estrogen levels fluctuate, influencing the menstrual cycle, bone density, and the health of reproductive organs.

During the reproductive years, estrogen is responsible for the development of secondary sexual characteristics, including breast development and the widening of hips. It also contributes to the thickening of the uterine lining in preparation for potential pregnancy. As women approach perimenopause and menopause, there is a gradual decline in estrogen levels, leading to changes in the menstrual cycle and various symptoms, such as hot flashes and mood swings.

Beyond its reproductive role, estrogen has broader implications for women's health, influencing cardiovascular health, bone density, and cognitive function. Maintaining a balance of estrogen is crucial for overall well-being, and disruptions in estrogen levels can contribute to conditions such as osteoporosis, heart disease, and cognitive decline.

Progesterone: The Protector of Pregnancy

Produced by the ovaries, progesterone is a hormone that works in tandem with estrogen to regulate the menstrual cycle and support pregnancy. During the menstrual cycle, progesterone levels rise following ovulation, preparing the uterine lining for potential implantation of a fertilized egg. If pregnancy does not occur, progesterone levels decrease, triggering the start of menstruation.

During pregnancy, the placenta takes over the role of producing progesterone, which is essential for maintaining the uterine lining and preventing contractions that could lead to preterm birth.

Progesterone also plays a role in breast development and the production of milk during breastfeeding.

In addition to its reproductive functions, progesterone has calming effects on the central nervous system. It can influence mood and sleep, and some women may experience changes in these aspects during the menstrual cycle.

Follicle-Stimulating Hormone (FSH) and Luteinizing Hormone (LH): Ovulation Orchestrators

FSH and LH are hormones produced by the pituitary gland that play a central role in the menstrual cycle and reproductive processes. FSH stimulates the development of follicles in the ovaries, each containing an egg. As the follicles mature, they produce estrogen.

LH, on the other hand, triggers ovulation—the release of a mature egg from the ovary. This surge in LH is a crucial event in the menstrual cycle, and it typically occurs around the midpoint of the cycle. After ovulation, the ruptured follicle transforms into a structure called the corpus luteum, which produces progesterone to support the potential implantation of a fertilized egg.

Monitoring FSH and LH levels is often used in fertility assessments and to understand the dynamics of the menstrual cycle. Elevated levels of these hormones can indicate conditions such as polycystic ovary syndrome (PCOS) or diminished ovarian reserve.

Testosterone: Beyond Masculinity

While often associated with male reproductive health, testosterone is also present in women, albeit in lower concentrations. Produced by the ovaries and adrenal glands, testosterone plays a role in supporting bone density, muscle mass, and libido in women.

In the ovaries, testosterone is converted to estrogen, highlighting the interconnected nature of these hormones. Low levels of testosterone can contribute to a decrease in libido, fatigue, and changes in mood. Disorders such as polycystic ovary syndrome (PCOS) can lead to elevated testosterone levels in women, affecting reproductive and metabolic health.

Balancing testosterone levels is essential for overall well-being, and healthcare professionals may consider hormonal interventions when imbalances are identified. It is important to recognize that testosterone contributes to various physiological functions in women beyond its commonly acknowledged role in male reproductive health.

Prolactin: The Milk Producer

Produced by the pituitary gland, prolactin is a hormone that plays a crucial role in breastfeeding. Its primary function is to stimulate the production of milk in the mammary glands after childbirth. Prolactin levels rise in response to the stimulation of the nipples during breastfeeding, reinforcing the milk production process.

While prolactin is essential for lactation, elevated levels outside of pregnancy and breastfeeding can indicate conditions such as hyperprolactinemia. This condition can disrupt menstrual cycles and fertility and may require medical evaluation and intervention.

Gonadotropin-Releasing Hormone (GnRH): Master Regulator

Produced by the hypothalamus, GnRH is a hormone that acts as the master regulator of the reproductive system. It stimulates the pituitary gland to release FSH and LH, initiating the menstrual cycle and governing the processes of ovulation and menstruation.

GnRH secretion is pulsatile, and its release is influenced by various factors, including stress, nutrition, and feedback from estrogen and progesterone. The delicate balance of GnRH pulsatility is crucial for the proper functioning of the menstrual cycle.

Disruptions in GnRH regulation can lead to irregular menstrual cycles, anovulation, and fertility issues. Understanding the role of GnRH provides insights into the intricate feedback loops that govern the female reproductive system.

Cortisol: The Stress Responder

Produced by the adrenal glands, cortisol is often known as the "stress hormone." While it is not specific to gender, cortisol plays a significant role in the overall health and well-being of women. In response to stress, cortisol mobilizes energy reserves, influences metabolism, and modulates the immune response.

Chronic stress can lead to dysregulation of cortisol levels, contributing to conditions such as adrenal fatigue and impacting reproductive health. Cortisol imbalances may influence the menstrual cycle, fertility, and the overall resilience of the body to stressors.

Balancing cortisol levels involves stress management strategies, including relaxation techniques, adequate sleep, and lifestyle modifications. Recognizing the impact of stress on hormonal health is crucial for supporting overall well-being.

Oxytocin: The Bonding Hormone

Produced by the hypothalamus and released by the pituitary gland, oxytocin is often referred to as the "love hormone" or "bonding hormone." It plays a crucial role in social bonding, emotional connections, and the rreproductiv processes.

Oxytocin is released in large quantities during activities such as childbirth and breastfeeding, fostering the mother-infant bond. It is also implicated in romantic relationships, promoting feelings of trust and attachment.

Beyond its role in reproductive processes, oxytocin contributes to stress reduction, social bonding, and overall emotional well-being. Understanding the multifaceted nature of oxytocin highlights its importance in the broader context of women's health.

Insulin: Blood Sugar Regulator

Produced by the pancreas, insulin is a hormone that regulates blood sugar levels. While not exclusive to women, insulin sensitivity and glucose metabolism are critical factors in women's health, particularly in the context of conditions like gestational diabetes and polycystic ovary syndrome (PCOS).

Insulin facilitates the uptake of glucose by cells, allowing them to use it for energy. Insulin resistance, a condition where cells become less responsive to insulin, can lead to elevated blood sugar levels and contribute to metabolic disorders.

Maintaining insulin sensitivity through a balanced diet, regular physical activity, and lifestyle modifications is crucial for preventing metabolic imbalances and supporting overall health.

Melatonin: The Sleep Regulator

Synthesized by the pineal gland, melatonin is a hormone that regulates the sleep-wake cycle. While not exclusive to women, melatonin levels can be influenced by hormonal changes, particularly during the menstrual cycle and menopause.

Melatonin production is influenced by exposure to light, with levels typically rising in the evening to promote sleep. Changes in melatonin levels may contribute to sleep disturbances and insomnia, especially during times of hormonal fluctuations.

Recognizing the role of melatonin in sleep regulation underscores the importance of healthy sleep patterns in supporting overall well-being, particularly in women experiencing hormonal transitions.

Thyroid Hormones: Metabolic Conductors

The thyroid hormones—thyroxine (T4) and triiodothyronine (T3)—play a crucial role in metabolism, energy regulation, and overall well-being. Produced by the thyroid gland, these hormones influence various physiological processes, including heart rate, body temperature, and the metabolism of nutrients.

Thyroid function is intricately linked to the female reproductive system, and imbalances in thyroid hormones can affect menstrual regularity, fertility, and pregnancy outcomes. Conditions such as hypothyroidism and hyperthyroidism require medical attention to restore hormonal balance and support overall health.

Understanding the interconnectedness of thyroid hormones with reproductive health highlights their significance in women's well-being.

Conclusion

The overview of key hormones in women provides a glimpse into the intricate hormonal landscape that governs reproductive processes, influences overall health, and contributes to the unique experiences of women throughout their lives. These hormones, each with its specific roles and functions, form an integrated network that responds to the dynamic changes within the female body.

From the orchestration of the menstrual cycle by estrogen and progesterone to the regulation of stress response by cortisol, and the bonding facilitated by oxytocin, these hormones work in concert to maintain balance and harmony. Recognizing the interplay between these hormones is essential for understanding women's health, from adolescence through the reproductive years and into the phases of perimenopause and menopause.

The delicate balance of hormones is susceptible to various factors, including lifestyle, stress, and medical conditions. As such, a holistic approach to women's health involves not only understanding the roles of these key hormones but also addressing factors that contribute to hormonal imbalances.

Empowering women with knowledge about their hormonal health is a crucial step in promoting overall well-being. It fosters informed decision-making, encourages proactive health management, and contributes to a deeper understanding of the interconnected nature of physiological processes.

In navigating the intricate terrain of hormonal changes, women can embrace the uniqueness of their experiences and work towards achieving hormonal balance through lifestyle choices, medical interventions when necessary, and a holistic approach to health. The overview of key hormones in women serves as a foundation for recognizing the profound influence of these chemical messengers on the intricate dance of life and well-being.

Role of Hormones in Women's Health

The human body is a complex and intricately designed system, where hormones play a pivotal role in regulating various physiological processes. In the context of women's health, hormones serve as the messengers that orchestrate the intricate dance of the menstrual cycle, guide reproductive processes, and influence overall well-being throughout different life stages. Understanding the profound role of hormones in women's health is essential for appreciating the interconnectedness of these biochemical signals with physical, emotional, and mental aspects of well-being.

The Menstrual Cycle and Reproductive Health

1. Estrogen: The Architect of Reproduction

Estrogen, a key player in women's health, is produced primarily by the ovaries. It holds a central role in the menstrual cycle, influencing the development of secondary sexual characteristics and supporting reproductive processes. Across the menstrual cycle, estrogen levels fluctuate, reaching their peak during the follicular phase, which precedes ovulation.

During the follicular phase, estrogen stimulates the development of ovarian follicles, each containing an egg. It also contributes to the thickening of the uterine lining in preparation for a potential pregnancy. Estrogen's influence extends beyond the reproductive system, impacting bone density, cardiovascular health, and cognitive function.

2. Progesterone: Nurturing the Uterine Environment

Produced by the ovaries and later by the corpus luteum after ovulation, progesterone complements the actions of estrogen in the menstrual cycle. Following ovulation, progesterone levels rise, preparing the uterine lining for the potential implantation of a fertilized egg. If pregnancy does not occur, progesterone levels decline, triggering menstruation.

Progesterone is not only crucial for the menstrual cycle but also plays a role in supporting pregnancy. During pregnancy, the placenta takes over progesterone production, ensuring the maintenance of the uterine lining and preventing contractions that could lead to preterm birth.

3. Follicle-Stimulating Hormone (FSH) and Luteinizing Hormone (LH): Ovulation Directors

The pituitary gland secretes FSH and LH, which play a central role in the regulation of the menstrual cycle. FSH stimulates the development of ovarian follicles, each containing an egg. As the follicles mature, they produce estrogen. LH, in turn, triggers ovulation—the release of a mature egg from the ovary.

This surge in LH is a critical event in the menstrual cycle, typically occurring around the midpoint. After ovulation, the ruptured follicle transforms into the corpus luteum, which produces progesterone. The delicate balance of FSH and LH is essential for the proper functioning of the reproductive system.

4. Gonadotropin-Releasing Hormone (GnRH): Master Regulator

GnRH, produced by the hypothalamus, serves as the master regulator of the menstrual cycle. It stimulates the pituitary gland to release FSH and LH, initiating the processes of ovulation and menstruation. The pulsatile secretion of GnRH is influenced by various factors, including stress, nutrition, and feedback from estrogen and progesterone.

Understanding the role of GnRH provides insights into the intricate feedback loops that govern the female reproductive system. Disruptions in GnRH regulation can lead to irregular menstrual cycles, anovulation, and fertility issues.

Pregnancy and Postpartum Period

1. Human Chorionic Gonadotropin (hCG): Sustaining Early Pregnancy

Produced by the placenta during pregnancy, hCG is a hormone that plays a crucial role in sustaining the early stages of pregnancy. It is the hormone detected by pregnancy tests and is responsible for maintaining the corpus luteum, which, in turn, produces progesterone to support the uterine lining.

hCG levels rise rapidly in the first weeks of pregnancy, providing a marker for the viability of the pregnancy. Understanding the role of hCG is essential for monitoring early pregnancy and ensuring the appropriate support for a developing fetus.

2. Prolactin: The Initiator of Milk Production

Produced by the pituitary gland, prolactin is a hormone that becomes prominent during pregnancy and the postpartum period. Its primary function is to stimulate the production of milk in the mammary glands after childbirth. Prolactin levels rise in response to the stimulation of the nipples during breastfeeding, initiating and sustaining the milk production process.

Prolactin is instrumental in establishing and maintaining breastfeeding, supporting the nutritional needs of the newborn. Elevated levels of prolactin outside of pregnancy and breastfeeding can indicate conditions such as hyperprolactinemia, which may require medical evaluation.

Menopause and Hormonal Transitions

1. Perimenopause: Navigating Hormonal Fluctuations

Perimenopause, the transitional phase leading to menopause, is characterized by hormonal fluctuations and changes in the menstrual cycle. Estrogen and progesterone levels may become irregular, leading to variations in the length and intensity of menstrual periods.

During perimenopause, women may experience symptoms such as hot flashes, night sweats, mood swings, and changes in libido. The understanding of hormonal changes during perimenopause is crucial for managing symptoms and supporting overall well-being.

2. Menopause: The Cessation of Menstruation

Menopause marks the end of the reproductive years, occurring when a woman has not had a menstrual period for 12 consecutive months. Estrogen and progesterone levels significantly decline during menopause, leading to a cessation of ovulation and menstruation.

The hormonal changes during menopause can have wide-ranging effects on various aspects of health, including bone density, cardiovascular health, and urogenital health. Managing hormonal transitions during menopause involves a holistic approach that considers lifestyle, nutrition, and, in some cases, hormone replacement therapy (HRT).

Hormones and Bone Health

1. Estrogen and Bone Density

Estrogen plays a crucial role in maintaining bone density. During the reproductive years, estrogen helps regulate the activity of osteoblasts (cells that build bone) and osteoclasts (cells that break down bone). The decline in estrogen levels during perimenopause and menopause contributes to accelerated bone loss, increasing the risk of osteoporosis.

Maintaining bone health involves strategies such as adequate calcium and vitamin D intake, weight-bearing exercises, and, in some cases, hormone replacement therapy (HRT) to mitigate the impact of estrogen decline on bone density.

Cardiovascular Health and Hormones

1. Estrogen and Cardiovascular Protection

Estrogen has cardioprotective effects, influencing cardiovascular health in premenopausal women. It contributes to the dilation of blood vessels, maintenance of healthy cholesterol levels, and overall vascular function. However, as estrogen levels decline during menopause, women become more susceptible to cardiovascular issues.

Postmenopausal women face an increased risk of conditions such as hypertension, elevated cholesterol levels, and atherosclerosis. Maintaining cardiovascular health after menopause involves lifestyle choices, including regular exercise, a heart-healthy diet, and, when appropriate, hormone replacement therapy (HRT).

Hormones and Mental Well-being

1. Estrogen and Cognitive Function

Estrogen receptors are present in various regions of the brain, indicating the hormone's influence on cognitive function and mood regulation. The decline in estrogen during menopause has been associated with changes in memory, concentration, and mood.

Hormone replacement therapy (HRT) has been explored as a potential intervention to support cognitive function in postmenopausal women. However, the decision to pursue HRT should be individualized, considering factors such as overall health and potential risks.

2. Hormones and Mood Regulation

Hormones play a significant role in mood regulation, and fluctuations in estrogen and progesterone levels throughout the menstrual cycle can impact mood. Some women may experience premenstrual mood changes, commonly known as premenstrual syndrome (PMS), due to hormonal variations.

Additionally, the hormonal transitions during perimenopause and menopause can contribute to mood swings, irritability, and an increased risk of depression and anxiety. Recognizing the influence of hormones on mental well-being is essential for comprehensive women's health care.

Hormones and Metabolic Health

1. Insulin Sensitivity and Hormones

Hormones, particularly insulin, play a critical role in metabolic health. Insulin facilitates the uptake of glucose by cells, allowing them to utilize it for energy. Insulin sensitivity, the ability of cells to respond to insulin, is essential for maintaining blood sugar levels within a healthy range.

Conditions such as gestational diabetes and polycystic ovary syndrome (PCOS) involve disruptions in insulin sensitivity. Managing metabolic health includes lifestyle modifications, such as a balanced diet and regular physical activity, to support insulin function.

Hormones and Sexual Health

While testosterone is often associated with male reproductive health, it also plays a role in women's sexual health. Produced by the ovaries and adrenal glands, testosterone influences libido, arousal, and overall sexual well-being in women.

Hormonal imbalances, such as low testosterone levels, can contribute to a decrease in sexual desire. Addressing sexual health involves a holistic approach that considers hormonal balance, psychological factors, and relationship dynamics.

Hormones and Sleep Regulation

Melatonin, produced by the pineal gland, regulates the sleep-wake cycle. Hormonal fluctuations, particularly during the menstrual cycle and menopause, can influence melatonin levels and impact sleep quality.

Recognizing the interplay between hormones and sleep regulation is crucial for addressing sleep disturbances in women. Strategies to support healthy sleep patterns include maintaining a consistent sleep schedule, creating a conducive sleep environment, and managing stress.

Hormones and Stress Response

Cortisol, often referred to as the "stress hormone," is produced by the adrenal glands and plays a crucial role in the body's response to stress. Chronic stress can lead to dysregulation of cortisol levels, impacting reproductive health, immune function, and overall resilience.

Managing stress involves adopting stress-reduction techniques, including mindfulness, relaxation exercises, and lifestyle modifications. Recognizing the impact of stress on hormonal health is vital for promoting overall well-being.

Hormones and the Immune System

Estrogen has been shown to influence immune function, with higher estrogen levels potentially enhancing the immune response. This may explain the observed differences in immune responses between men and women. However, the relationship between hormones and immune function is complex and involves various factors.

Hormonal fluctuations during the menstrual cycle and hormonal changes in menopause can influence immune responses. Understanding the interplay between hormones and the immune system contributes to a holistic approach to women's health.

Conclusion

In summary, hormones are the silent conductors of the intricate symphony that is women's health. From the onset of puberty through the reproductive years and into the phases of perimenopause and menopause, hormones shape the unique experiences of women. They influence reproductive

processes, bone health, cardiovascular function, mental well-being, and various aspects of overall health.

Recognizing the profound role of hormones in women's health is not only crucial for understanding the intricacies of the female body but also for empowering women to make informed decisions about their well-being. A holistic approach to women's health involves considering the interconnectedness of hormonal, physical, emotional, and mental aspects.

As advancements in medical research continue to unveil the complexities of hormonal regulation, healthcare providers can tailor interventions to support women at different stages of life. Whether addressing reproductive health, managing hormonal transitions, or promoting overall well-being, a comprehensive understanding of the role of hormones lays the foundation for personalized and effective healthcare strategies.

As women navigate the dynamic landscape of their hormonal journey, informed choices, regular health check-ups, and a proactive approach to well-being can contribute to a fulfilling and empowered life. The role of hormones in women's health is not just a biological phenomenon but a testament to the resilience, strength, and beauty inherent in every woman's journey.

CHAPTER THREE
Common Symptoms of Hormonal Imbalances

Hormones are intricate messengers that orchestrate a myriad of physiological processes in the human body. When these delicate chemical signals fall out of balance, the effects can manifest in various ways, giving rise to a range of symptoms. Hormonal imbalances can affect both men and women, impacting different stages of life and contributing to a host of health issues. In this comprehensive exploration, we delve into the common symptoms of hormonal imbalances, shedding light on how these disruptions can manifest across different systems and aspects of well-being.

Reproductive System Symptoms

1. Irregular Menstrual Cycles: Hormonal imbalances often manifest in irregular menstrual cycles for women. Fluctuations in estrogen and progesterone levels can lead to unpredictable or absent periods. Conditions such as polycystic ovary syndrome (PCOS) or thyroid disorders can contribute to menstrual irregularities, highlighting the intricate interplay between hormones.

2. Heavy or Painful Periods: Hormonal imbalances may result in abnormal uterine bleeding, leading to heavy or prolonged periods. Estrogen dominance or insufficient progesterone levels can disrupt the normal menstrual flow, causing discomfort and potential complications.

3. Premenstrual Syndrome (PMS): Changes in hormonal levels during the menstrual cycle can contribute to premenstrual symptoms. Emotional changes, bloating, breast tenderness, and mood swings are common manifestations of hormonal fluctuations in the days leading up to menstruation.

4. Hot Flashes and Night Sweats: Menopausal women often experience hot flashes and night sweats, which are attributed to declining estrogen levels. These sudden sensations of heat can be disruptive to sleep and daily activities, impacting the quality of life for women going through menopause.

5. Vaginal Dryness: Estrogen plays a crucial role in maintaining the health of vaginal tissues. A decline in estrogen levels, particularly during menopause, can lead to vaginal dryness, discomfort during intercourse, and an increased risk of urinary tract infections.

6. Changes in Libido: Hormonal imbalances, especially involving testosterone, can impact libido in both men and women. Low levels of testosterone may contribute to a decreased interest in sexual activity, affecting relationships and overall well-being.

Metabolic and Weight-Related Symptoms

1. Weight Gain or Difficulty Losing Weight: Hormonal imbalances, such as insulin resistance or thyroid disorders, can contribute to weight gain or difficulty losing weight. Insulin resistance, in particular, may lead to increased fat storage and metabolic dysfunction.

2. Increased Belly Fat: Elevated cortisol levels, often associated with chronic stress, can contribute to the accumulation of abdominal or visceral fat. This type of fat is linked to an increased risk of cardiovascular disease and metabolic disorders.

3. Changes in Appetite: Hormonal imbalances may influence appetite regulation, leading to changes in eating patterns. For instance, imbalances in leptin and ghrelin, known as the "hunger hormones," can contribute to overeating or difficulty maintaining a healthy weight.

Skin and Hair Symptoms

1. Acne or Breakouts: Hormonal imbalances, particularly fluctuations in androgens like testosterone, can contribute to the development of acne. Adult-onset acne in women may be indicative of hormonal disruptions, requiring targeted interventions for effective management.

2. Excessive Hair Growth or Hair Loss: Conditions such as polycystic ovary syndrome (PCOS) can lead to elevated levels of androgens, resulting in hirsutism or excessive hair growth in areas

where men typically grow hair. On the flip side, hormonal imbalances can also contribute to hair loss, a common concern in both men and women.

3. Changes in Skin Tone and Texture: Estrogen and collagen production are closely linked, and a decline in estrogen levels can contribute to changes in skin tone and texture. Reduced collagen may lead to the development of fine lines, wrinkles, and sagging skin.

Mood and Mental Health Symptoms

1. Mood Swings: Hormonal fluctuations, especially during the menstrual cycle, perimenopause, and menopause, can contribute to mood swings. Changes in estrogen and progesterone levels may impact neurotransmitters in the brain, influencing mood and emotional well-being.

2. Anxiety and Depression: Hormones play a significant role in mental health, and imbalances can contribute to symptoms of anxiety and depression. Postpartum hormonal shifts, thyroid disorders, and fluctuations in sex hormones are among the factors linked to mood disorders.

3. Irritability and Agitation: Hormonal imbalances, particularly involving cortisol and adrenal hormones, can contribute to feelings of irritability and agitation. Chronic stress, which affects hormonal regulation, is often associated with these symptoms.

4. Difficulty Concentrating: Hormonal imbalances can influence cognitive function and concentration. Changes in estrogen levels, particularly during perimenopause and menopause, may contribute to forgetfulness and difficulty focusing.

Sleep-Related Symptoms

1. Insomnia: Hormonal imbalances, particularly those affecting melatonin production, can contribute to difficulty falling asleep or staying asleep. Sleep disturbances may be more pronounced during times of hormonal fluctuations, such as the menstrual cycle or menopause.

2. Fatigue: Disruptions in cortisol levels, often associated with chronic stress or adrenal imbalances, can contribute to fatigue. Hormonal imbalances affecting thyroid function may also lead to persistent feelings of tiredness.

Cardiovascular Symptoms

1. Irregular Heartbeat: Thyroid hormones play a crucial role in cardiovascular function, and imbalances can contribute to irregular heartbeats or palpitations. Hyperthyroidism, characterized by excess thyroid hormone, is often associated with an increased heart rate.

2. Changes in Blood Pressure: Hormonal imbalances may influence blood pressure regulation. Conditions such as adrenal disorders can contribute to fluctuations in blood pressure, impacting cardiovascular health.

Digestive System Symptoms

1. Bloating and Digestive Discomfort: Hormonal imbalances, particularly those affecting progesterone levels, can contribute to bloating and digestive discomfort. These symptoms are commonly experienced during the premenstrual phase.

2. Changes in Appetite and Cravings: Hormonal fluctuations may influence appetite and food cravings. For example, changes in insulin sensitivity can lead to increased cravings for sugary or carbohydrate-rich foods.

Immune System Symptoms

Hormonal imbalances can impact immune function, potentially leading to increased susceptibility to infections. Estrogen, in particular, has been shown to influence immune responses, and fluctuations in estrogen levels may affect the body's ability to fend off pathogens.

Musculoskeletal Symptoms

Hormonal imbalances, particularly those involving estrogen, can contribute to joint pain and stiffness. Some women may experience exacerbation of symptoms during the menstrual cycle or menopause.

In conclusion, the symptoms of hormonal imbalances are diverse and can affect various systems within the body. From reproductive health and metabolism to mental well-being and cardiovascular function, hormones play a pervasive role in maintaining balance and harmony. Recognizing the signs of hormonal imbalances is the first step towards seeking appropriate interventions and improving overall health.

It's important to note that individual responses to hormonal fluctuations can vary, and the severity of symptoms may differ from person to person. Seeking guidance from healthcare professionals is crucial for accurate diagnosis and tailored treatment plans. Whether addressing hormonal imbalances through lifestyle modifications, hormone replacement therapy, or other interventions, a holistic approach to well-being is key to restoring equilibrium and promoting health at every stage of life.

Recognizing Patterns and Triggers of Hormonal Imbalance

Hormonal balance is a delicate and intricate aspect of a woman's overall health, influencing various physiological processes from puberty through menopause. The endocrine system, comprised of glands that produce hormones, plays a crucial role in maintaining this delicate equilibrium. However, numerous factors, both internal and external, can disrupt this balance, leading to hormonal imbalances. Recognizing the patterns and triggers of hormonal imbalance is essential for women to understand their bodies, manage their health proactively, and seek appropriate interventions when necessary.

Before delving into patterns and triggers of hormonal imbalance, it's crucial to understand the endocrine system's fundamental role in the body. The endocrine system consists of glands—such as the pituitary, thyroid, adrenal, and ovaries—that release hormones into the bloodstream. These hormones act as messengers, coordinating various functions, including metabolism, growth, immune response, and reproduction.

The hypothalamus, located in the brain, serves as the master regulator, orchestrating the release of hormones from the pituitary gland. The pituitary gland, in turn, signals other glands to release specific hormones. For example, the thyroid gland produces thyroid hormones, the adrenal glands release cortisol, and the ovaries produce estrogen and progesterone.

Hormonal Patterns Across the Menstrual Cycle

The menstrual cycle provides a natural framework to observe hormonal patterns in women. Understanding the phases of the menstrual cycle—menstruation, the follicular phase, ovulation, and the luteal phase—offers insights into the dynamic interplay of hormones.

1. Menstruation: The menstrual cycle begins with menstruation, marked by the shedding of the uterine lining. During this phase, estrogen and progesterone levels are low. The decrease in hormones triggers the release of follicle-stimulating hormone (FSH) from the pituitary gland, initiating the development of ovarian follicles.

2. Follicular Phase:As the menstrual cycle progresses, rising levels of estrogen stimulate the growth of ovarian follicles. This phase culminates in a surge of luteinizing hormone (LH), triggering ovulation. The follicular phase is characterized by increasing estrogen levels, reaching their peak just before ovulation.

3. Ovulation: Ovulation marks the release of a mature egg from the ovary. Estrogen levels peak during this phase, contributing to the surge in LH. After ovulation, the ruptured follicle transforms into the corpus luteum, which produces progesterone.

4. Luteal Phase: The luteal phase is characterized by elevated progesterone levels, preparing the uterine lining for potential implantation. If fertilization does not occur, the corpus luteum breaks down, and estrogen and progesterone levels decline, leading to the onset of menstruation.

Common Patterns of Hormonal Imbalance

1. Estrogen Dominance: Estrogen dominance occurs when there is an excess of estrogen relative to progesterone. This imbalance can result from factors such as stress, diet, or impaired liver function, which affects estrogen metabolism. Symptoms may include heavy or irregular periods, breast tenderness, and mood swings.

2. Progesterone Deficiency:In contrast, a deficiency in progesterone relative to estrogen can lead to hormonal imbalance. This may result in symptoms such as irregular periods, mood swings, anxiety, and difficulty maintaining pregnancies. Conditions like polycystic ovary syndrome (PCOS) can contribute to progesterone deficiency.

3. Thyroid Imbalances: The thyroid gland produces hormones (T3 and T4) that regulate metabolism. Thyroid imbalances, such as hypothyroidism (underactive thyroid) or hyperthyroidism (overactive thyroid), can disrupt the menstrual cycle, lead to weight changes, and affect energy levels.

4. Adrenal Fatigue: The adrenal glands, located atop the kidneys, release hormones like cortisol in response to stress. Chronic stress can lead to adrenal fatigue, disrupting cortisol levels. Symptoms may include fatigue, sleep disturbances, and hormonal imbalances affecting the menstrual cycle.

5. Insulin Resistance: Insulin, a hormone produced by the pancreas, regulates blood sugar levels. Insulin resistance occurs when cells become less responsive to insulin, leading to elevated blood sugar levels. This can contribute to conditions like polycystic ovary syndrome (PCOS) and disrupt hormonal balance.

6. Cortisol Dysregulation: Chronic stress can lead to dysregulation of cortisol, the primary stress hormone. Elevated cortisol levels over time can impact the menstrual cycle, contribute to weight gain, and affect sleep. Cortisol dysregulation is often associated with adrenal fatigue.

Common Triggers of Hormonal Imbalance

1. Chronic Stress: Chronic stress is a significant trigger for hormonal imbalance. The body's response to stress involves the release of cortisol, which, when prolonged, can disrupt the balance of other hormones, including those involved in the menstrual cycle.

2. Poor Nutrition: Diet plays a crucial role in hormonal health. Nutrient deficiencies, imbalances in macronutrients, and excessive consumption of processed foods can impact hormone production and function. Poor nutrition can contribute to conditions like insulin resistance and thyroid imbalances.

3. Lack of Physical Activity: Sedentary lifestyles can contribute to hormonal imbalances, particularly those related to insulin sensitivity and metabolism. Regular physical activity is essential for maintaining hormonal balance and supporting overall health.

4. Endocrine-Disrupting Chemicals: Exposure to endocrine-disrupting chemicals (EDCs) in the environment can interfere with hormone function. EDCs, found in certain pesticides, plastics, and pollutants, may mimic or block hormones, leading to imbalances.

5. Unhealthy Sleep Habits: Sleep is crucial for hormonal regulation, particularly melatonin and cortisol. Disruptions in the sleep-wake cycle or inadequate sleep can affect hormone production, leading to imbalances that impact various bodily functions.

6. Menopause and Aging: The natural aging process, especially during menopause, involves a decline in estrogen and progesterone levels. This hormonal shift can lead to various symptoms, emphasizing the need for women to adapt to the changes and seek support if necessary.

7. Medical Conditions: Certain medical conditions, such as polycystic ovary syndrome (PCOS), thyroid disorders, and diabetes, can contribute to hormonal imbalances. Managing these conditions is crucial for restoring hormonal equilibrium.

8. Medications and Birth Control: Some medications, including hormonal contraceptives, can influence hormone levels. Changes in birth control methods or certain medications may impact hormonal balance, requiring adjustments and monitoring.

Recognizing Signs of Hormonal Imbalance

1. Changes in Menstrual Cycle: Irregularities in the menstrual cycle, such as missed periods, heavy bleeding, or significant changes in flow, may indicate hormonal imbalance.

2. Mood Swings and Emotional Changes: Fluctuations in hormones can affect mood. Women experiencing unexplained mood swings, anxiety, or depression should consider hormonal factors.

3. Sleep Disturbances: Hormonal imbalances can disrupt sleep patterns. Insomnia, difficulty falling or staying asleep, or changes in sleep quality may signal hormonal issues.

4. Changes in Skin and Hair: Hormonal imbalances can impact skin and hair health. Acne, excessive hair growth, or hair loss may be indicative of underlying hormonal issues.

5. Weight Changes: Sudden weight gain or difficulty losing weight despite efforts may be linked to hormonal imbalances affecting metabolism.

6. Fatigue and Energy Levels: Persistent fatigue or changes in energy levels unrelated to sleep patterns may be a sign of hormonal disruption, especially cortisol dysregulation.

7. Reproductive Health Issues: Fertility challenges, recurrent miscarriages, or difficulties conceiving may indicate hormonal imbalances affecting reproductive health.

8. Digestive Issues: Hormonal imbalances can influence digestive health, leading to symptoms such as bloating, changes in appetite, or gastrointestinal discomfort.

Seeking Professional Guidance

While recognizing patterns and triggers of hormonal imbalance is valuable, seeking professional guidance is essential for accurate diagnosis and personalized treatment. Healthcare providers, including gynecologists, endocrinologists, and naturopathic doctors, can conduct thorough evaluations, including hormone testing, to identify imbalances.

Conclusion

Recognizing patterns and triggers of hormonal imbalance empowers women to take an active role in their health. By understanding the natural fluctuations in hormonal levels, identifying signs of imbalance, and addressing contributing factors, women can make informed choices to support their well-being.

It's important to approach hormonal health holistically, considering lifestyle factors, stress management, and professional guidance. Regular check-ups, open communication with healthcare providers, and a proactive attitude toward health contribute to maintaining hormonal balance throughout different stages of life. As women navigate the dynamic landscape of their hormonal journey, awareness, education, and personalized care play pivotal roles in fostering overall well-being.

CHAPTER FOUR

Nutrition for Hormonal Health

Nutrition plays a pivotal role in maintaining hormonal health in women throughout various stages of life. The delicate interplay of hormones regulates reproductive functions, metabolism, mood, and overall well-being. An optimal diet that provides essential nutrients supports hormonal balance and helps mitigate the risk of imbalances that can lead to a range of health issues. In this comprehensive exploration, we delve into the impact of nutrition on hormonal health, the key nutrients involved, and dietary strategies that women can adopt to promote hormonal equilibrium.

The Impact of Nutrition on Hormonal Health:

1. Macronutrients:

Proteins:

- Essential for hormone production, proteins provide amino acids necessary for synthesizing hormones like estrogen and insulin.

- Sources include lean meats, poultry, fish, dairy, legumes, and plant-based proteins.

Fats:

- Healthy fats, such as omega-3 and omega-6 fatty acids, are precursors to hormone production.

- Fatty fish, flaxseeds, chia seeds, avocados, and nuts are rich in these essential fats.

Carbohydrates:

- Complex carbohydrates provide sustained energy and support serotonin production, influencing mood.

- Whole grains, fruits, vegetables, and legumes are excellent sources of complex carbohydrates.

2. Micronutrients:

Vitamins:

Vitamin D:

- Essential for hormone regulation, including estrogen and progesterone.

- Sunlight exposure, fatty fish, fortified foods, and supplements contribute to vitamin D levels.

Vitamin B6:

- Involved in estrogen metabolism and serotonin production.

- Found in poultry, fish, bananas, potatoes, and fortified cereals.

Vitamin E:

- Acts as an antioxidant, supporting overall hormonal health.

- Nuts, seeds, spinach, and broccoli are good sources of vitamin E.

<u>**Minerals:**</u>

Calcium:

- Critical for bone health and plays a role in hormonal regulation.

- Dairy products, leafy greens, and fortified plant-based milk are calcium sources.

Iron:

- Essential for transporting oxygen and supporting energy metabolism.

- Red meat, beans, lentils, and fortified cereals are iron-rich foods.

Zinc:

- Supports immune function and plays a role in hormone production.

- Found in meat, dairy, nuts, and legumes.

Selenium:

- Acts as an antioxidant and supports thyroid function.

- Selenium-rich foods include Brazil nuts, fish, and poultry.

3. Phytoestrogens:

- Plant compounds with estrogen-like properties that may help balance hormonal levels.

- Found in soy products, flaxseeds, lentils, and whole grains.

4. Fiber:

- Supports digestive health and helps eliminate excess hormones from the body.

- Fruits, vegetables, whole grains, and legumes are excellent sources of fiber.

5. Antioxidants:

- Protect cells from oxidative stress and support overall health.

- Berries, dark leafy greens, nuts, and colorful vegetables are rich in antioxidants.

Dietary Strategies for Hormonal Health:

1. Balanced Diet:

- Prioritize a diverse and balanced diet that includes a variety of fruits, vegetables, whole grains, lean proteins, and healthy fats.

- Avoid excessive intake of processed foods, refined sugars, and trans fats.

2. Adequate Protein Intake:

- Include protein-rich foods in each meal to support hormone synthesis and overall health.

- Options include lean meats, fish, dairy, eggs, legumes, and plant-based proteins.

3. Healthy Fats:

- Incorporate sources of healthy fats, such as avocados, fatty fish, nuts, seeds, and olive oil.

- Omega-3 fatty acids, in particular, are crucial for hormonal health.

4. Fiber-Rich Foods:

- Consume a variety of fiber-rich foods to support digestive health and hormone elimination.

- Choose whole grains, fruits, vegetables, and legumes.

5. Phytoestrogen-Rich Foods:

- Include phytoestrogen-rich foods like soy products, flaxseeds, lentils, and whole grains in the diet.

- These foods may help modulate estrogen levels.

6. Hydration:

- Ensure adequate hydration, as water is essential for overall health and hormonal balance.

- Limit the intake of sugary beverages and excessive caffeine.

7. Vitamin and Mineral-Rich Foods:

   - Consume a variety of foods rich in vitamins and minerals, including fruits, vegetables, nuts, seeds, and lean proteins.

   - Consider supplementation if specific nutrient needs are not met through diet alone.

8. Limit Processed Foods and Sugar:

   - Reduce the intake of processed foods, refined sugars, and artificial additives, which can contribute to hormonal imbalances.

   - Opt for whole, nutrient-dense foods.

9. Manage Stress:

   - Incorporate stress-reducing activities such as meditation, yoga, deep breathing, and regular physical exercise.

   - Chronic stress can disrupt hormonal balance, so managing stress is crucial.

10. Regular Physical Activity:

   - Engage in regular exercise to support overall health and hormonal balance.

   - Both aerobic and strength-training exercises contribute to well-being.

11. Mindful Eating:

   - Practice mindful eating by paying attention to hunger and fullness cues.

   - This approach promotes a healthy relationship with food and supports hormonal regulation.

12. Individualized Approach:

   - Recognize that individual nutritional needs vary, and it's essential to tailor dietary choices based on factors like age, activity level, and specific health conditions.

Conclusion:

Nutrition plays a fundamental role in supporting hormonal health in women. A well-balanced and nutrient-rich diet contributes to the synthesis and regulation of hormones that influence reproductive health, metabolism, mood, and overall well-being. By prioritizing key nutrients, incorporating a variety of foods, and adopting healthy dietary strategies, women can empower themselves to maintain hormonal equilibrium throughout different stages of life.

It's important to note that individual nutritional needs may vary, and consulting with healthcare professionals or registered dietitians can provide personalized guidance. By adopting a holistic approach to nutrition, women can proactively support their hormonal health and enhance their overall quality of life.

Lifestyle Changes and Stress Management

The intricate dance of hormones in a woman's body influences various aspects of her health, from reproductive functions and metabolism to mood and overall well-being. Hormonal imbalances can arise due to a myriad of factors, and lifestyle choices play a crucial role in either exacerbating or mitigating these imbalances. In this comprehensive exploration, we delve into the impact of lifestyle changes and stress management on hormone repair in women. By understanding the connections between lifestyle, stress, and hormonal health, women can empower themselves to make informed choices that support hormonal equilibrium.

The Interplay of Lifestyle and Hormonal Health:

1. Nutrition:

Balanced Diet:

- A well-balanced diet is foundational for hormone repair. Nutrient-rich foods provide the building blocks for hormone synthesis and regulation.

- Include a variety of fruits, vegetables, whole grains, lean proteins, and healthy fats in your diet.

Impact of Macronutrients:

- Adequate protein intake supports the production of hormones like estrogen and insulin.

- Healthy fats, such as omega-3 fatty acids, are essential for hormonal balance.

- Complex carbohydrates provide sustained energy and influence serotonin production, affecting mood.

Hydration:

- Staying adequately hydrated is crucial for overall health and hormonal balance.

- Limit the consumption of sugary beverages and prioritize water intake.

Phytoestrogen-Rich Foods:

- Incorporate foods rich in phytoestrogens, such as soy products, flaxseeds, and legumes, to support estrogen balance.

Limit Processed Foods:

- Reduce the intake of processed foods, refined sugars, and artificial additives, as they can contribute to hormonal imbalances.

2. Physical Activity:

Exercise for Hormonal Health:

- Regular physical activity contributes to hormonal balance by improving insulin sensitivity and supporting overall metabolic health.

- Both aerobic exercises and strength training play a role in maintaining well-being.

Weight Management:

- Maintaining a healthy weight is essential for hormonal health. Excess body fat, especially around the abdomen, can contribute to hormonal imbalances.

- Engage in activities you enjoy to make exercise a sustainable part of your lifestyle.

Mind-Body Practices:

- Practices like yoga and tai chi not only provide physical activity but also promote stress reduction, supporting hormonal balance.

3. Stress Management:

The Impact of Chronic Stress:

- Chronic stress can disrupt the delicate balance of hormones, leading to imbalances in cortisol, estrogen, and other key hormones.

- The adrenal glands, which produce stress hormones like cortisol, may become overworked with chronic stress.

Mindfulness and Meditation:

- Incorporate mindfulness and meditation practices into your routine to reduce stress levels.

- Mindful breathing, guided meditation, and progressive muscle relaxation are effective techniques.

Yoga and Relaxation Techniques:

- Yoga combines physical activity with stress-reducing techniques. It has been shown to lower cortisol levels and improve overall well-being.

- Relaxation techniques, such as deep breathing and visualization, can be practiced regularly.

Establishing Boundaries:

- Setting clear boundaries in personal and professional life is crucial for managing stress.

- Learn to say no when necessary and prioritize self-care.

Social Support:

- Maintaining strong social connections provides emotional support, which can buffer the impact of stress on hormonal health.

- Foster relationships with friends, family, and support groups.

4. Sleep Hygiene:

The Importance of Sleep:

- Quality sleep is essential for hormonal repair and overall well-being.

- Lack of sleep or poor sleep quality can disrupt the circadian rhythm, affecting hormones like melatonin and cortisol.

Establishing Healthy Sleep Habits:

- Maintain a consistent sleep schedule by going to bed and waking up at the same time each day.

- Create a sleep-conducive environment with minimal light and noise.

Screen Time and Blue Light:

- Limit exposure to electronic devices before bedtime, as the blue light emitted can interfere with melatonin production.

- Consider blue light filters on devices or using "night mode" settings.

Hormone Repair Strategies at Different Life Stages:

1. Adolescence and Puberty:

Nutrition and Balanced Diet:

- Provide essential nutrients during this crucial developmental stage to support the onset of menstruation.

- Educate young women about the importance of a balanced diet for hormonal health.

Physical Activity and Body Image:

- Encourage regular physical activity to support hormonal balance and promote a positive body image.

- Emphasize the importance of a healthy approach to weight management.

Stress Management Techniques:

- Introduce stress management techniques early on to help adolescents cope with academic and social pressures.

- Foster open communication about stressors and emotional well-being.

2. Reproductive Years:

Balancing Hormones During Menstrual Cycle:

- Women can track their menstrual cycles and observe patterns in hormonal fluctuations.

- Understanding the phases of the menstrual cycle helps women anticipate and manage hormonal changes.

Nutrient-Rich Diet for Fertility:

- For women trying to conceive, a nutrient-rich diet supports fertility and hormonal balance.

- Adequate intake of folic acid, iron, and other essential nutrients is crucial.

Stress Reduction for Fertility:

- Chronic stress can impact fertility. Implement stress reduction techniques to support reproductive health.

- Consider mind-body approaches such as acupuncture or fertility-focused yoga.

3. Perimenopause and Menopause:

Hormonal Changes and Symptom Management:

- Understand the hormonal shifts during perimenopause and menopause.

- Manage symptoms such as hot flashes, mood swings, and sleep disturbances through lifestyle and, if necessary, medical interventions.

Bone Health:

- Adequate calcium and vitamin D intake become particularly important during menopause to support bone health.

- Weight-bearing exercises contribute to bone density.

Stress Reduction for Hormonal Harmony:

- Stress management is crucial during perimenopause and menopause, as stress can exacerbate symptoms.

- Mindfulness, meditation, and relaxation techniques are beneficial.

Hormone Replacement Therapy (HRT):

- Discuss the potential benefits and risks of hormone replacement therapy with healthcare providers.

- HRT can be considered for managing severe symptoms, but it's not suitable for everyone.

Holistic Approaches to Hormone Repair:

1. Mind-Body Connection:

Psychoneuroimmunology:

- The field of psychoneuroimmunology explores the interconnectedness of the mind, nervous system, and immune system.

- Emotions and stress can impact immune function and hormonal balance.

Mindful Eating:

- Adopt a mindful approach to eating, paying attention to hunger and fullness cues.

- Mindful eating promotes a healthy relationship with food and supports hormonal regulation.

2. Environmental Factors:

Endocrine Disruptors:

- Be aware of endocrine-disrupting chemicals (EDCs) in the environment.

- Reduce exposure to EDCs by choosing organic products, using glass or stainless steel containers, and avoiding certain plastics.

Household and Personal Care Products:

- Check the ingredients of household and personal care products for potential endocrine disruptors.

- Opt for products with fewer synthetic chemicals.

Seeking Professional Guidance:

1. Regular Check-ups:

- Schedule regular check-ups with healthcare providers, including gynecologists and endocrinologists.

- Discuss hormonal health and any concerns or symptoms experienced.

2. Hormone Testing:

- If hormonal imbalances are suspected, healthcare providers may recommend hormone testing.

- Hormone levels can provide valuable insights into the underlying causes of symptoms.

3. Individualized Treatment Plans:

- Work with healthcare providers to develop individualized treatment plans.

- Treatment may include lifestyle modifications, nutritional interventions, medications, or hormone therapy, depending on the specific situation.

Conclusion:

Hormone repair in women is a multifaceted journey that involves making conscious lifestyle choices and effectively managing stress. By understanding the interconnectedness of nutrition, physical activity, stress management, and hormonal health, women can embark on a path toward greater well-being. From adolescence through reproductive years and into menopause, adopting holistic approaches that address the unique needs of each life stage contributes to sustained hormonal balance.

Empowering women with knowledge about their bodies and the tools to support hormone repair fosters a proactive approach to health. By embracing lifestyle changes, managing stress effectively, and seeking professional guidance when needed, women can navigate the intricate landscape of hormonal health with resilience and vitality. As a result, they can cultivate a sense of harmony and well-being that extends beyond hormonal balance, encompassing the entirety of their physical, emotional, and mental health.

Exercise for Hormone Balance

Exercise is a powerful and versatile tool that plays a crucial role in maintaining overall health and well-being. In women, physical activity has a profound impact on hormonal balance, influencing the intricate interplay of hormones that regulate various physiological functions. From reproductive health to mood and metabolism, exercise can positively modulate hormone levels, promoting equilibrium throughout different stages of life. In this comprehensive exploration, we delve into the specific ways in which exercise contributes to hormone balance in women, the types of exercises that are most beneficial, and how incorporating regular physical activity into one's lifestyle can enhance overall health.

Exercise and Estrogen Balance:

1. Regular Menstrual Cycle:

   - Regular menstrual cycles are indicative of a balanced hormonal environment.

   - Physical activity, when moderate and consistent, contributes to regular menstrual cycles by promoting overall health.

2. Impact of Intense Exercise:

   - Intense and prolonged exercise, such as that seen in competitive athletes, can lead to disruptions in the menstrual cycle.

   - This is often referred to as exercise-induced amenorrhea and is associated with low estrogen levels.

3. Moderate Exercise and Estrogen:

   - Moderate-intensity exercise has been shown to have a positive impact on estrogen levels.

- Weight-bearing exercises, such as walking, jogging, and resistance training, contribute to bone health and estrogen balance.

4. Bone Health:

- Estrogen plays a crucial role in maintaining bone density. Reduced estrogen levels, as seen in menopause, are associated with bone loss.

- Weight-bearing and resistance exercises support bone health by stimulating bone formation.

Exercise and Progesterone Balance:

1. Luteal Phase Support:

- Progesterone levels rise during the luteal phase of the menstrual cycle.

- Regular exercise can support progesterone balance by promoting overall reproductive health.

2. Stress Management:

- Chronic stress can contribute to progesterone deficiency.

- Exercise acts as a stress-reducing activity, positively influencing cortisol levels and supporting progesterone balance.

Testosterone and Exercise:

1. Lean Body Mass and Testosterone:

- Testosterone plays a role in maintaining lean body mass and muscle function.

- Resistance training, in particular, stimulates the release of testosterone, contributing to muscle growth and repair.

2. High-Intensity Exercise:

- High-intensity interval training (HIIT) has been shown to increase testosterone levels.

- Short bursts of intense exercise followed by rest periods can be an effective strategy.

Insulin Sensitivity and Metabolic Health:

1. Role of Insulin:

   - Insulin sensitivity is crucial for maintaining stable blood sugar levels and preventing insulin resistance.

   - Regular physical activity, especially aerobic exercise, improves insulin sensitivity.

2. Cardiovascular Exercise:

   - Cardiovascular exercises such as running, cycling, and swimming enhance insulin sensitivity.

   - These activities help regulate blood sugar levels and support metabolic health.

Cortisol Regulation through Exercise:

1. Exercise as a Stress Regulator:

   - Exercise acts as a natural stress regulator, helping to manage cortisol levels.

   - Regular physical activity, especially activities like yoga and moderate-intensity exercise, promotes stress resilience.

2. Timing of Exercise:

   - The timing of exercise can influence cortisol levels. Morning exercise can help regulate cortisol rhythms and contribute to a healthy stress response.

Thyroid Hormones and Exercise:

1. Role of Thyroid Hormones:

   - Thyroid hormones regulate metabolism and energy production.

   - Regular exercise supports thyroid function by promoting overall metabolic health.

2. Impact of Overtraining:

   - Intense and prolonged exercise, especially without adequate recovery, can negatively impact thyroid function.

   - Balancing exercise intensity with proper rest is crucial for thyroid health.

Growth Hormone Release and Resistance Training:

1. Stimulating Growth Hormone:

   - Resistance training, including weightlifting and bodyweight exercises, stimulates the release of growth hormone.

   - Growth hormone is essential for muscle growth, repair, and overall vitality.

2. Timing and Intensity:

   - Performing resistance exercises with adequate intensity and incorporating them into a well-rounded fitness routine maximizes growth hormone release.

Tailoring Exercise for Different Life Stages:

1. Adolescence and Puberty:

   - Introduce a variety of physical activities to support overall health and development.

   - Emphasize the importance of a positive body image and healthy exercise habits.

2. Reproductive Years:

   - Choose exercises that align with reproductive goals, whether it's supporting fertility or maintaining overall well-being.

   - Incorporate a mix of cardiovascular, strength, and flexibility exercises.

3. Perimenopause and Menopause:

   - Adjust exercise routines to accommodate changes in bone density, muscle mass, and metabolic rate.

   - Focus on activities that promote bone health, such as weight-bearing exercises.

Balancing Cardiovascular and Strength Training:

1. Cardiovascular Exercise:

   - Cardiovascular activities, such as running, cycling, and swimming, support heart health and metabolic balance.

- Aim for at least 150 minutes of moderate-intensity or 75 minutes of vigorous-intensity aerobic exercise per week.

2. Strength Training:

- Resistance training, including weightlifting and bodyweight exercises, is crucial for maintaining muscle mass and supporting hormonal health.

- Include strength training at least two days per week, targeting major muscle groups.

Holistic Approaches to Hormone-Balancing Exercise:

1. Mind-Body Practices:

- Incorporate mind-body practices such as yoga and tai chi into the exercise routine.

- These practices not only enhance flexibility and strength but also promote stress reduction.

2. Consistency and Moderation:

- Consistency is key when it comes to exercise for hormone balance.

- Avoid extremes in exercise intensity or duration, as overtraining can lead to hormonal imbalances.

3. Individualized Approach:

- Recognize that individual responses to exercise may vary.

- Tailor exercise routines to personal preferences, fitness levels, and health goals.

Seeking Professional Guidance:

1. Consulting Healthcare Providers:

- Before embarking on a new exercise routine, especially for individuals with existing health conditions, consult with healthcare providers.

- Discussing exercise plans with healthcare professionals ensures safety and appropriateness.

2. Hormone Testing:

- In cases of suspected hormonal imbalances, hormone testing may provide valuable insights.

- Healthcare providers can interpret test results and guide individuals toward appropriate interventions.

Conclusion:

Exercise stands as a cornerstone in the pursuit of hormonal balance for women. By understanding the intricate relationship between physical activity and hormonal health, women can tailor their exercise routines to support overall well-being. Whether aiming to regulate estrogen and progesterone, boost testosterone, improve insulin sensitivity, or manage stress, exercise offers a versatile and accessible means to promote hormonal equilibrium.

Through a balanced and individualized approach to exercise that incorporates cardiovascular activities, strength training, and mind-body practices, women can harness the benefits of physical activity at every stage of life. Embracing a holistic perspective that considers the interplay of hormones, nutrition, and lifestyle factors empowers women to take charge of their health and cultivate a sense of vitality and balance that extends beyond the realm of exercise, influencing the entirety of their physical, emotional, and hormonal well-being.

CHAPTER FIVE

Nutrient-Rich Meal Plans

Nutrition plays a pivotal role in hormonal balance, influencing various physiological functions in women throughout different life stages. A well-crafted and nutrient-rich meal plan provides the essential building blocks for hormone synthesis, supports metabolic processes, and contributes to overall health and well-being. In this comprehensive exploration, we delve into the key nutrients that impact hormonal balance in women, the role of a balanced diet in supporting hormonal health, and specific nutrient-rich meal plans tailored to promote optimal hormone balance.

Key Nutrients for Hormone Balance:

1. Proteins:

 - Proteins are crucial for hormone synthesis, providing the necessary amino acids.

 - Include lean sources of protein such as poultry, fish, tofu, legumes, and dairy in meals.

2. Healthy Fats:

- Essential fatty acids, especially omega-3 and omega-6, are precursors to hormone production.

- Incorporate sources of healthy fats like fatty fish, flaxseeds, chia seeds, avocados, and nuts into the diet.

3. Complex Carbohydrates:

- Complex carbohydrates provide sustained energy and influence serotonin production.

- Include whole grains, fruits, vegetables, and legumes for a rich source of complex carbohydrates.

4. Vitamins:

- Vitamin D:

- Essential for hormonal regulation, including estrogen and progesterone.

- Sunlight exposure, fatty fish, fortified foods, and supplements contribute to vitamin D levels.

- Vitamin B6:

- Involved in estrogen metabolism and serotonin production.

- Found in poultry, fish, bananas, potatoes, and fortified cereals.

- Vitamin E:

- Acts as an antioxidant, supporting overall hormonal health.

- Nuts, seeds, spinach, and broccoli are good sources of vitamin E.

5. Minerals:

- Calcium:

- Critical for bone health and plays a role in hormonal regulation.

- Dairy products, leafy greens, and fortified plant-based milk are calcium sources.

- Iron:

- Essential for transporting oxygen and supporting energy metabolism.

- Red meat, beans, lentils, and fortified cereals are iron-rich foods.

- Zinc:

- Supports immune function and plays a role in hormone production.

- Found in meat, dairy, nuts, and legumes.

- Selenium:

  - Acts as an antioxidant and supports thyroid function.

  - Selenium-rich foods include Brazil nuts, fish, and poultry.

6. Phytoestrogens:

  - Plant compounds with estrogen-like properties that may help balance hormonal levels.

  - Found in soy products, flaxseeds, lentils, and whole grains.

7. Fiber:

  - Supports digestive health and helps eliminate excess hormones from the body.

  - Fruits, vegetables, whole grains, and legumes are excellent sources of fiber.

8. Antioxidants:

  - Protect cells from oxidative stress and support overall health.

  - Berries, dark leafy greens, nuts, and colorful vegetables are rich in antioxidants.

Balancing Macronutrients in Hormone-Balancing Meal Plans:

1. Breakfast: Quinoa and Berry Bowl:

  - Ingredients:

  - 1 cup cooked quinoa

  - Mixed berries (blueberries, strawberries, raspberries)

  - Chopped nuts (walnuts, almonds)

  - Greek yogurt

  - Honey for sweetness

  - Instructions:

  - Combine cooked quinoa with mixed berries.

  - Top with chopped nuts for healthy fats and a source of protein.

  - Add a dollop of Greek yogurt for additional protein and creaminess.

- Drizzle with honey for sweetness.

- **Nutritional Benefits:**

  - Quinoa provides complex carbohydrates, protein, and essential amino acids.

  - Berries contribute antioxidants and fiber.

  - Nuts offer healthy fats, protein, and micronutrients.

  - Greek yogurt is a source of probiotics and additional protein.

2. Lunch: Salmon and Avocado Salad:

- **Ingredients:**

  - Grilled or baked salmon fillet

  - Mixed greens (spinach, kale, arugula)

  - Cherry tomatoes

  - Avocado slices

  - Quinoa or brown rice

  - Olive oil and balsamic vinegar for dressing

- **Instructions:**

  - Arrange mixed greens on a plate.

  - Top with grilled or baked salmon.

  - Add cherry tomatoes and avocado slices.

  - Incorporate cooked quinoa or brown rice for complex carbohydrates.

  - Drizzle with olive oil and balsamic vinegar for a healthy dressing.

- **Nutritional Benefits:**

  - Salmon provides omega-3 fatty acids and protein.

  - Leafy greens offer fiber, vitamins, and minerals.

  - Avocado contributes healthy fats and potassium.

  - Quinoa or brown rice provides complex carbohydrates.

3. Snack: Greek Yogurt Parfait:

- **Ingredients:**

  - Greek yogurt

  - Mixed berries

  - Granola (preferably low in added sugars)

  - Chia seeds

- **Instructions:**

  - In a glass or bowl, layer Greek yogurt with mixed berries.

  - Add a layer of granola for crunch and additional carbohydrates.

  - Sprinkle chia seeds on top for added fiber and omega-3 fatty acids.

- **Nutritional Benefits:**

  - Greek yogurt provides protein and probiotics.

  - Berries offer antioxidants and fiber.

  - Granola adds complex carbohydrates.

  - Chia seeds contribute omega-3 fatty acids and fiber.

4. Dinner: Lentil and Vegetable Stir-Fry:

- **Ingredients:**

  - Cooked lentils

  - Mixed vegetables (broccoli, bell peppers, snap peas)

  - Tofu or tempeh for plant-based protein

  - Brown rice or quinoa

  - Soy sauce and sesame oil for seasoning

- **Instructions:**

  - Stir-fry mixed vegetables in a pan with tofu or tempeh.

  - Add cooked lentils for additional protein and fiber.

  - Serve over brown rice or quinoa.

  - Season with soy sauce and a drizzle of sesame oil.

- **Nutritional Benefits:**

  - Lentils provide protein and fiber.

  - Mixed vegetables offer vitamins and minerals.

  - Tofu or tempeh contributes plant-based protein.

  - Brown rice or quinoa provides complex carbohydrates.

Delicious and Hormone-Supportive Recipes

Creating delicious meals that also support hormonal balance is an empowering and enjoyable way for women to take charge of their health. A nutrient-rich and well-balanced diet is crucial for promoting hormonal equilibrium, and incorporating flavorful, hormone-supportive recipes into daily meals adds both variety and satisfaction to one's culinary experience. In this exploration, we will delve into a collection of delicious recipes that focus on key nutrients and food groups known for their positive impact on hormonal health. These recipes are designed to cater to different tastes and dietary preferences while providing essential nutrients for women's well-being.

Omega-3 Rich Salmon Salad Bowl:

Ingredients:

- 1 cup quinoa, cooked

- 1 medium-sized salmon fillet, grilled or baked

- Mixed greens (spinach, arugula, and kale)

- 1/2 avocado, sliced

- Cherry tomatoes, halved

- 1/4 cup walnuts, chopped

- Lemon-tahini dressing:

  - 2 tablespoons tahini

  - Juice of 1 lemon

  - 1 tablespoon olive oil

  - Salt and pepper to taste

Instructions:

1. In a bowl, assemble the cooked quinoa as the base.

2. Top with mixed greens, cherry tomatoes, sliced avocado, and grilled salmon.

3. Sprinkle chopped walnuts over the salad.

4. In a small bowl, whisk together tahini, lemon juice, olive oil, salt, and pepper to create the dressing.

5. Drizzle the dressing over the salad just before serving.

Hormone-Balancing Berry Smoothie Bowl:

Ingredients:

- 1 cup mixed berries (blueberries, strawberries, raspberries)

- 1 banana, frozen

- 1/2 cup Greek yogurt

- 1 tablespoon chia seeds

- 1 tablespoon almond butter

- Granola for topping

Instructions:

1. In a blender, combine mixed berries, frozen banana, Greek yogurt, chia seeds, and almond butter.

2. Blend until smooth and creamy.

3. Pour the smoothie into a bowl.

4. Top with granola for added crunch and texture.

5. Garnish with additional berries and a dollop of Greek yogurt if desired.

Quinoa and Chickpea Power Bowl:

Ingredients:

- 1 cup cooked quinoa

- 1 cup cooked chickpeas

- 1 cup cherry tomatoes, halved

- 1 cucumber, diced

- 1/4 cup feta cheese, crumbled

- Kalamata olives, pitted

- Fresh parsley, chopped

- Lemon-olive oil dressing:

  - 2 tablespoons extra-virgin olive oil

  - Juice of 1 lemon

  - 1 clove garlic, minced

  - Salt and pepper to taste

Instructions:

1. In a bowl, combine cooked quinoa, chickpeas, cherry tomatoes, diced cucumber, feta cheese, and olives.

2. In a small jar, shake together olive oil, lemon juice, minced garlic, salt, and pepper to create the dressing.

3. Drizzle the dressing over the quinoa and chickpea mixture.

4. Toss the salad gently to combine.

5. Garnish with fresh parsley before serving.

Stir-Fried Tofu and Vegetable Quinoa Bowl:

Ingredients:

- 1 cup cooked quinoa

- 1 block firm tofu, cubed

- Broccoli florets

- Bell peppers, thinly sliced

- Carrots, julienned

- Snap peas

- 2 tablespoons soy sauce

- 1 tablespoon sesame oil

- 1 tablespoon rice vinegar

- 1 teaspoon ginger, grated

- 2 cloves garlic, minced

- Sesame seeds for garnish

Instructions:

1. In a large skillet, sauté cubed tofu until golden brown.

2. Add broccoli, bell peppers, carrots, and snap peas to the skillet.

3. In a small bowl, whisk together soy sauce, sesame oil, rice vinegar, grated ginger, and minced garlic.

4. Pour the sauce over the tofu and vegetables, stirring to coat evenly.

5. Serve the stir-fried tofu and vegetables over a bed of cooked quinoa.

6. Garnish with sesame seeds for added flavor and texture.

Hormone-Supportive Green Goddess Smoothie:

Ingredients:

- 1 cup kale, stems removed

- 1/2 cucumber, peeled and sliced

- 1 green apple, cored and diced

- 1/2 lemon, peeled

- 1 tablespoon flaxseeds

- 1 tablespoon almond butter

- 1 cup coconut water

- Ice cubes (optional)

Instructions:

1. In a blender, combine kale, cucumber, green apple, lemon, flaxseeds, almond butter, and coconut water.

2. Blend until smooth and creamy.

3. Add ice cubes if a colder temperature is desired.

4. Pour the green goddess smoothie into a glass and enjoy.

Sweet Potato and Black Bean Enchiladas:

Ingredients:

- 2 medium-sized sweet potatoes, peeled and diced

- 1 can black beans, drained and rinsed

- 1 cup corn kernels (fresh or frozen)

- 1 teaspoon cumin

- 1 teaspoon chili powder

- 1/2 teaspoon smoked paprika

- 1/2 teaspoon garlic powder

- 8 whole-grain tortillas

- Enchilada sauce (store-bought or homemade)

- 1 cup shredded cheese (cheddar or Mexican blend)

- Fresh cilantro for garnish

Instructions:

1. Preheat the oven to 375°F (190°C).

2. Steam or roast the diced sweet potatoes until tender.

3. In a large bowl, mash the sweet potatoes and mix with black beans, corn, cumin, chili powder, smoked paprika, and garlic powder.

4. Spoon the sweet potato and black bean mixture onto each tortilla, roll them up, and place them seam-side down in a baking dish.

5. Pour enchilada sauce over the rolled tortillas, ensuring they are well-covered.

6. Sprinkle shredded cheese over the top.

7. Bake in the preheated oven for 20-25 minutes or until the cheese is melted and bubbly.

8. Garnish with fresh cilantro before serving.

Mediterranean Quinoa Salad:

Ingredients:

- 1 cup cooked quinoa

- Cherry tomatoes, halved

- Cucumber, diced

- Kalamata olives, pitted and sliced

- Red onion, finely chopped

- Feta cheese, crumbled

- Fresh parsley, chopped

- Lemon-oregano dressing:

  - 2 tablespoons extra-virgin olive oil

  - Juice of 1 lemon

  - 1 teaspoon dried oregano

  - Salt and pepper to taste

Instructions:

1. In a bowl, combine cooked quinoa, cherry tomatoes, diced cucumber, sliced Kalamata olives, chopped red onion, and crumbled feta cheese.

2. In a small jar, shake together olive oil, lemon juice, dried oregano, salt, and pepper to create the dressing.

3. Drizzle the dressing over the quinoa salad and toss gently to combine.

4. Garnish with fresh parsley before serving.

Chocolate Avocado Mousse:

Ingredients:

- 2 ripe avocados, peeled and pitted

- 1/4 cup unsweetened cocoa powder

- 1/4 cup maple syrup or honey

- 1 teaspoon vanilla extract

- Pinch of salt

- Berries for topping

Instructions:

1. In a food processor, blend together avocados, cocoa powder, maple syrup (or honey), vanilla extract, and a pinch of salt.

2. Blend until the mixture is smooth and creamy.

3. Spoon the chocolate avocado mousse into serving glasses.

4. Chill in the refrigerator for at least 30 minutes.

5. Top with fresh berries before serving.

Turmeric-Ginger Golden Milk Latte:

Ingredients:

- 1 cup unsweetened almond milk

- 1 teaspoon ground turmeric

- 1/2 teaspoon ground ginger

- 1 tablespoon honey or maple syrup

- 1/2 teaspoon vanilla extract

- Pinch of black pepper

Instructions:

1. In a small saucepan, heat almond milk over medium heat.

2. Whisk in ground turmeric, ground ginger, honey (or maple syrup), vanilla extract, and a pinch of black pepper.

3. Continue to whisk until the mixture is heated but not boiling.

4. Pour the golden milk into a mug and enjoy.

Roasted Vegetable and Quinoa Stuffed Bell Peppers:

Ingredients:

- 4 bell peppers, halved and seeds removed

- 1 cup cooked quinoa

- Mixed vegetables (zucchini, cherry tomatoes, red onion, mushrooms), diced

- 1 cup black beans, cooked

- 1 teaspoon cumin

- 1 teaspoon smoked paprika

- 1/2 teaspoon garlic powder

- Olive oil

- Fresh cilantro for garnish

Instructions:

1. Preheat the oven to 375°F (190°C).

2. In a bowl, mix cooked quinoa, diced mixed vegetables, black beans, cumin, smoked paprika, and garlic powder.

3. Drizzle olive oil over the bell peppers and stuff each half with the quinoa and vegetable mixture.

4. Place the stuffed bell peppers in a baking dish.

5. Bake in the preheated oven for 25-30 minutes or until the peppers are tender.

6. Garnish with fresh cilantro before serving.

Incorporating these delicious and hormone-supportive recipes into your culinary repertoire not only enhances the flavors of your meals but also contributes to a well-balanced and nutrient-rich diet. By prioritizing key nutrients, such as omega-3 fatty acids, proteins, vitamins, minerals, and phytoestrogens, these recipes are designed to support hormonal balance at different stages of a woman's life.

Experiment with these recipes, modify them to suit your taste preferences, and enjoy the journey of nourishing your body with wholesome and flavorful foods. Remember that a varied and colorful diet not only supports hormonal health but also contributes to overall well-being, fostering a sense of vitality and balance in your daily life.

CHAPTER SIX

Overview of Herbal Remedies

Hormonal balance is crucial for the overall health and well-being of women. Hormones play a vital role in regulating various physiological functions, including the menstrual cycle, mood, metabolism, and reproductive health. Imbalances in hormone levels can lead to a range of symptoms and health issues. While conventional medical treatments are available, many women also explore alternative approaches, such as herbal remedies, to address hormonal imbalances. In this comprehensive overview, we will explore various herbs that have been traditionally used to promote hormonal balance in women, their potential benefits, and considerations for incorporating herbal remedies into a holistic approach to women's health.

Key Herbal Remedies for Hormonal Imbalance:

1. Chaste Tree Berry (Vitex agnus-castus):

   - Also known as Vitex, chaste tree berry is one of the most popular herbs for women's hormonal health.

   - It is believed to support the balance of estrogen and progesterone and is commonly used to alleviate symptoms of premenstrual syndrome (PMS), irregular menstrual cycles, and breast tenderness.

2. Black Cohosh (Actaea racemosa):

   - Black cohosh has a long history of use in Native American medicine and is often recommended for menopausal symptoms.

   - It is believed to have estrogenic effects and may help reduce hot flashes, night sweats, and mood swings associated with menopause.

3. Red Clover (Trifolium pratense):

   - Red clover contains compounds known as isoflavones, which have estrogen-like effects.

   - It is commonly used to alleviate menopausal symptoms and may also support bone health.

4. Dong Quai (Angelica sinensis):

   - Dong Quai, also known as "female ginseng," is a traditional Chinese herb used to support women's reproductive health.

   - It is believed to regulate estrogen levels and is often used for menstrual irregularities and menopausal symptoms.

5. Maca Root (Lepidium meyenii):

- Maca root, native to the Andes Mountains, is an adaptogenic herb known for its potential to balance hormones.

- It is often used to support energy, stamina, and reproductive health, especially during periods of hormonal changes.

6. Ashwagandha (Withania somnifera):

- Ashwagandha is an adaptogenic herb with a wide range of health benefits.

- It may help modulate cortisol levels, reduce stress, and support overall hormonal balance, making it beneficial for women experiencing stress-related hormonal issues.

7. Wild Yam (Dioscorea villosa):

- Wild yam has been traditionally used to support women's reproductive health.

- While it doesn't contain hormones, it is believed to have estrogen-like effects and is used for menstrual issues and menopausal symptoms.

8. Rhodiola (Rhodiola rosea):

- Rhodiola is an adaptogenic herb that may help the body adapt to stress.

- It is believed to influence cortisol levels and may indirectly support hormonal balance by reducing stress-related impacts on the endocrine system.

9. Licorice Root (Glycyrrhiza glabra):

- Licorice root is known for its sweet taste and has been used in traditional medicine for various purposes.

- It may have mild estrogenic effects and is sometimes used to address hormonal imbalances, particularly in the adrenal glands.

10. Saw Palmetto (Serenoa repens):

- Saw palmetto is often associated with prostate health in men, but it may also have benefits for women.

- It is believed to modulate hormones and is sometimes used to address symptoms associated with polycystic ovary syndrome (PCOS).

Considerations and Precautions:

While herbal remedies can offer potential benefits, it's essential to approach their use with caution and under the guidance of a healthcare professional. Consider the following points:

1. Individual Variability:

   - Responses to herbal remedies can vary widely among individuals.

   - What works well for one person may not be suitable for another, and dosage requirements may differ.

2. Quality and Standardization:

   - The quality of herbal supplements can vary, and it's crucial to choose products from reputable manufacturers.

   - Look for standardized extracts to ensure consistent potency.

3. Interactions with Medications:

   - Herbal remedies may interact with medications, affecting their effectiveness or causing unwanted side effects.

   - Consult with a healthcare provider, especially if you are taking prescription medications.

4. Pregnancy and Breastfeeding:

   - Some herbs may not be safe during pregnancy or breastfeeding.

   - It's essential for pregnant or breastfeeding women to consult with a healthcare professional before using herbal remedies.

5. Potential Side Effects:

   - While herbal remedies are generally considered safe, they can still have side effects.

   - Monitor for any adverse reactions and discontinue use if necessary.

6. Timing and Duration of Use:

   - The timing and duration of herbal remedy use may vary based on individual needs and goals.

   - Short-term or intermittent use may be recommended for certain herbs.

Integrating Herbal Remedies into a Holistic Approach:

1. Consultation with Healthcare Provider:

   - Before incorporating herbal remedies, consult with a healthcare provider, preferably one with expertise in herbal medicine.

   - Discuss your symptoms, health history, and any ongoing treatments.

2. Holistic Lifestyle Approaches:

   - Herbal remedies work best when integrated into a holistic approach that includes a balanced diet, regular exercise, stress management, and adequate sleep.

   - Addressing lifestyle factors can contribute significantly to hormonal balance.

3. Trial and Observation:

   - Begin with a cautious approach, especially if trying a new herbal remedy.

   - Start with a lower dosage and observe how your body responds before considering adjustments.

4. Regular Monitoring:

   - Regularly monitor your symptoms and overall well-being.

   - Be open to adjusting your herbal regimen based on changes in symptoms or overall health.

5. Combination of Herbs:

   - Some women find that a combination of herbs works synergistically to address multiple aspects of hormonal balance.

   - However, it's crucial to approach combinations thoughtfully and with professional guidance.

6. Educate Yourself:

   - Take the time to educate yourself about the herbs you are considering.

   - Understand their mechanisms of action, potential side effects, and any contraindications.

Herbal remedies have been an integral part of traditional medicine systems worldwide, offering a holistic and natural approach to addressing various health concerns, including hormonal imbalances in women. While scientific research on the efficacy of herbal remedies for hormonal balance continues, many women report positive experiences with certain herbs.

It's essential to approach the use of herbal remedies with a well-informed and cautious mindset. Consulting with a healthcare provider who has expertise in herbal medicine can provide personalized guidance based on individual health needs and considerations. Integrating herbal remedies into a holistic lifestyle approach that includes proper nutrition, exercise, and stress management can contribute to overall well-being and hormonal balance in women.

Alternative Therapies for Hormonal Health

Maintaining hormonal health is integral to a woman's overall well-being, influencing various aspects of physical and mental health throughout different stages of life. While conventional medical approaches play a crucial role in managing hormonal imbalances, many women are exploring alternative therapies as complementary options to support their hormonal health. In this comprehensive overview, we will delve into various alternative therapies, including acupuncture, yoga, aromatherapy, and mindfulness practices, to understand their potential benefits for women's hormonal balance.

Acupuncture for Hormonal Balance:

Acupuncture, an ancient Chinese medicine practice, involves the insertion of thin needles into specific points on the body. It is based on the concept of energy flow, or Qi, and aims to restore balance to the body's energy pathways. In the context of women's health, acupuncture has shown promise in addressing hormonal imbalances associated with menstrual irregularities, fertility issues, and menopausal symptoms.

Mechanisms of Action:

1. Regulating Hormone Levels:

   - Acupuncture is believed to influence the endocrine system, including the hypothalamus, pituitary gland, and ovaries.

   - By stimulating specific acupuncture points, it may help regulate the secretion of hormones such as estrogen and progesterone.

2. Reducing Stress and Cortisol Levels:

- Chronic stress can contribute to hormonal imbalances in women.

- Acupuncture has been shown to promote relaxation, reduce stress levels, and modulate the release of cortisol, thereby supporting hormonal balance.

3. Improving Blood Flow:

- Enhanced blood circulation through acupuncture may contribute to better ovarian function and the regulation of menstrual cycles.

- Improved blood flow may also benefit women experiencing fertility issues.

Application:

1. Menstrual Irregularities:

- Acupuncture may be considered for women with irregular menstrual cycles or conditions such as polycystic ovary syndrome (PCOS).

- Regular acupuncture sessions may help regulate menstrual flow and alleviate associated symptoms.

2. Fertility Support:

- Some women undergoing fertility treatments may choose acupuncture as a complementary therapy.

- It is often used to support reproductive health, enhance blood flow to the uterus, and reduce stress related to fertility challenges.

3. Menopausal Symptoms:

- Acupuncture has been explored as a non-pharmacological option for managing menopausal symptoms such as hot flashes, mood swings, and sleep disturbances.

- Regular acupuncture sessions may offer relief for some women experiencing these symptoms.

Yoga for Hormonal Balance:

Yoga, an ancient practice originating from India, encompasses physical postures, breath control, meditation, and ethical principles. It is known for its holistic approach to health, addressing not only the physical body but also mental and emotional well-being. In the realm of women's health, yoga is considered a beneficial alternative therapy for promoting hormonal balance across various life stages.

Mechanisms of Action:

1. Stress Reduction:

  - Chronic stress can disrupt hormonal balance, affecting the menstrual cycle and reproductive health.

  - Yoga, with its emphasis on mindfulness and relaxation, can help reduce stress levels and mitigate the impact on hormones.

2. Physical Exercise and Endorphin Release:

  - Regular practice of yoga involves physical movement and poses that stimulate the endocrine system.

  - Physical activity, combined with the meditative aspects of yoga, can lead to the release of endorphins, which contribute to a sense of well-being.

3. Improved Circulation:

  - Certain yoga poses are designed to enhance blood circulation, particularly in the pelvic area.

  - Improved blood flow can support ovarian function, regulate menstrual cycles, and contribute to reproductive health.

Application:

1. Menstrual Health:

  - Women experiencing irregular menstrual cycles or conditions like PCOS may find yoga beneficial.

  - Gentle yoga practices that focus on breath awareness and relaxation can be particularly helpful.

2. Fertility Support:

  - Yoga is often recommended as a complementary therapy for women undergoing fertility treatments.

  - Fertility-focused yoga sequences may include poses that promote pelvic circulation and reduce stress.

3. Menopausal Symptoms:

  - Yoga can offer relief from common menopausal symptoms, including hot flashes, mood swings, and insomnia.

- Restorative and yin yoga, in particular, may be soothing for women navigating the menopausal transition.

Aromatherapy for Hormonal Well-being:

Aromatherapy involves the use of essential oils extracted from plants to promote physical, emotional, and psychological well-being. The inhalation or topical application of these oils is believed to stimulate the olfactory system and impact various physiological processes. In the context of women's hormonal health, specific essential oils are thought to have properties that can help balance hormones, reduce stress, and alleviate symptoms related to menstruation and menopause.

Mechanisms of Action:

1. Impact on the Limbic System:

   - The olfactory system is closely connected to the limbic system, which plays a role in emotions, mood, and hormonal regulation.

   - Inhaling certain essential oils is believed to influence the limbic system and, consequently, hormonal balance.

2. Stress Reduction:

   - Aromatherapy is often used as a relaxation technique, contributing to stress reduction.

   - Reduced stress levels can positively impact hormonal health, especially in relation to the menstrual cycle.

3. Potential Phytoestrogenic Effects:

   - Some essential oils, such as clary sage and fennel, are considered to have phytoestrogenic properties.

   - These oils may interact with estrogen receptors in the body, potentially influencing hormonal balance.

Application:

1. Menstrual Symptoms:

   - Essential oils like clary sage and lavender are commonly used to alleviate symptoms associated with menstruation, including cramps and mood swings.

   - Aromatherapy through diffusers or diluted oils in massage may provide relief.

2. Menopausal Symptoms:

- Women experiencing hot flashes, night sweats, and mood changes during menopause may benefit from aromatherapy.

- Essential oils like peppermint, lemon, and geranium are often recommended for their cooling and balancing effects.

3. Stress Management:

- Aromatherapy can be integrated into stress management practices.

- Oils such as lavender, chamomile, and bergamot are known for their calming properties and can be diffused or used in massages.

Mindfulness and Meditation for Hormonal Harmony:

Mindfulness and meditation practices involve cultivating present-moment awareness and a non-judgmental attitude toward thoughts and emotions. These practices, rooted in contemplative traditions, have gained recognition for their positive impact on mental health, stress reduction, and overall well-being. In the context of hormonal health, mindfulness and meditation are valued for their ability to modulate the stress response and promote a sense of balance.

Mechanisms of Action:

1. Stress Reduction:

- Chronic stress can contribute to hormonal imbalances in women.

- Mindfulness practices, including meditation, have been shown to reduce stress and promote relaxation, indirectly supporting hormonal harmony.

2. Cortisol Regulation:

- Mindfulness practices may influence cortisol levels, the primary stress hormone.

- By modulating cortisol, mindfulness may have downstream effects on other hormones, contributing to a more balanced hormonal profile.

3. Improved Emotional Regulation:

- Hormones and emotions are interconnected, and emotional well-being plays a role in hormonal health.

- Mindfulness and meditation practices enhance emotional regulation, potentially positively impacting hormonal balance.

Application:

1. Menstrual Health:

   - Women experiencing symptoms such as mood swings, irritability, or emotional fluctuations during the menstrual cycle may find mindfulness beneficial.

   - Regular mindfulness practices can foster emotional resilience.

2. Fertility Support:

   - Mindfulness practices can be valuable for women navigating fertility challenges.

   - They offer a supportive framework for managing stress associated with fertility treatments.

3. Menopausal Symptoms:

   - Mindfulness and meditation can be incorporated into the management of menopausal symptoms.

   - By promoting relaxation and emotional balance, these practices may alleviate symptoms such as anxiety and sleep disturbances.

Herbal Teas for Hormonal Support:

In addition to incorporating specific herbs into one's diet, herbal teas can be a delightful and practical way to enjoy the benefits of medicinal plants. Certain herbs are known for their potential to support hormonal balance, ease menstrual discomfort, and provide relaxation. While not a replacement for medical treatment, herbal teas can be a comforting addition to a woman's routine.

Popular Herbal Teas for Hormonal Support:

1. Raspberry Leaf Tea:

   - Raspberry leaf is traditionally used to support women's reproductive health.

   - It is believed to tone the uterine muscles and may be consumed throughout various stages of a woman's life.

2. Chamomile Tea:

   - Chamomile has calming properties and is often used to promote relaxation and alleviate stress.

   - It can be beneficial for women experiencing sleep disturbances or anxiety.

3. Nettle Tea:

- Nettle is rich in nutrients, including iron and calcium.

- It is sometimes used to support overall health, including during menstruation and menopause.

4. Peppermint Tea:

- Peppermint tea has a refreshing flavor and is known for its digestive benefits.

- It may be soothing for women experiencing menstrual cramps.

5. Ginger Tea:

- Ginger has anti-inflammatory properties and may help alleviate menstrual cramps.

- It is also valued for its warming effect.

6. Dandelion Root Tea:

- Dandelion root is thought to support liver health, which plays a role in hormone metabolism.

- It is often consumed as a detoxifying tea.

Considerations and Precautions:

While alternative therapies can offer valuable support for hormonal health, it's essential to approach them mindfully and in consultation with healthcare professionals, particularly for women with existing health conditions or those undergoing medical treatments. Consider the following points:

1. Individualized Approach:

- The effectiveness of alternative therapies can vary among individuals.

- It's crucial to adopt an individualized approach, considering personal health history, preferences, and responses to specific therapies.

2. Integration with Conventional Care:

- Alternative therapies should be seen as complementary to, not a replacement for, conventional medical care.

- Inform healthcare providers about any alternative therapies being pursued.

3. Professional Guidance:

- Seek guidance from qualified practitioners or experts in the respective alternative therapies.

- Professionals can provide personalized recommendations based on individual health needs.

4. Safety and Quality:

   - Ensure the safety and quality of products used in alternative therapies, such as essential oils or herbal supplements.

   - Choose reputable brands and, when applicable, consult with herbalists or aromatherapists.

5. Monitoring and Adaptation:

   - Regularly monitor the effects of alternative therapies on symptoms and overall well-being.

   - Be open to adaptations in the approach based on individual responses.

6. Pregnancy and Breastfeeding:

   - Women who are pregnant or breastfeeding should exercise caution and consult with healthcare providers before using certain herbs or engaging in specific therapies.

7. Mind-Body Connection:

   - Recognize the interconnectedness of the mind and body.

   - Practices that promote mental and emotional well-being can contribute positively to hormonal health.

Conclusion:

Alternative therapies for hormonal health provide women with a diverse set of tools to support their well-being. From ancient practices like acupuncture and yoga to modern approaches like aromatherapy and mindfulness, these therapies offer holistic avenues to address hormonal imbalances and enhance overall health.

Individual preferences, health goals, and responses to various therapies can vary, emphasizing the importance of an individualized approach. By integrating alternative therapies with conventional care and seeking guidance from qualified practitioners, women can empower themselves to actively participate in their health journey.

Whether it's the calming effects of a yoga session, the soothing aroma of essential oils, the mindful embrace of meditation, or the nourishing properties of herbal teas, these alternative therapies contribute to a comprehensive approach to hormonal health. Through informed choices and a commitment to holistic well-being, women can navigate the intricate landscape of hormonal balance with greater resilience and vitality.

CHAPTER SEVEN

The Importance of Regular Hormone Checks for Women's Health

Hormones play a crucial role in regulating various physiological functions in the body, influencing everything from metabolism and mood to reproductive health. For women, hormonal balance is particularly important throughout different stages of life, from adolescence to menopause. Regular hormone checks, which involve assessing the levels of key hormones in the body, are vital for maintaining overall health and well-being. In this comprehensive exploration, we will delve into the significance of regular hormone checks, the key hormones that are commonly assessed, and the benefits of early detection and intervention in addressing hormonal imbalances.

The Importance of Hormonal Balance:

Maintaining hormonal balance is essential for overall health and well-being. Hormones act in a delicate interplay, and even small imbalances can have profound effects on physical and mental health. Common factors that can contribute to hormonal imbalances in women include:

1. Puberty: The onset of puberty brings significant hormonal changes as estrogen and progesterone levels rise, leading to the development of secondary sexual characteristics.

2. Menstrual Cycle: Fluctuations in estrogen and progesterone levels during the menstrual cycle can lead to symptoms such as mood swings, bloating, and changes in energy levels.

3. Pregnancy: Hormonal changes during pregnancy are essential for fetal development but can also result in symptoms like morning sickness and mood swings.

4. Perimenopause and Menopause: As women approach menopause, estrogen and progesterone levels decline, leading to symptoms such as hot flashes, mood changes, and changes in bone density.

5. Medical Conditions: Conditions such as polycystic ovary syndrome (PCOS), thyroid disorders, and diabetes can disrupt hormonal balance.

6. Stress: Chronic stress can impact cortisol levels, affecting the balance of other hormones and contributing to a range of health issues.

The Significance of Regular Hormone Checks:

Regular hormone checks involve assessing the levels of specific hormones through blood, urine, or saliva tests. These checks provide valuable information about the functioning of the endocrine system and can help identify hormonal imbalances or abnormalities early on. The significance of regular hormone checks for women's health can be understood through various perspectives:

1. Early Detection of Hormonal Imbalances:

   - Regular hormone checks allow for the early detection of hormonal imbalances, providing an opportunity for timely intervention.

   - Early detection is particularly crucial for conditions such as PCOS, thyroid disorders, and hormonal cancers.

2. Monitoring Reproductive Health:

   - For women trying to conceive, hormone checks can provide insights into reproductive health.

   - Assessing levels of estrogen, progesterone, and other fertility-related hormones helps identify factors that may impact fertility.

3. Management of Menopausal Symptoms:

   - During perimenopause and menopause, hormonal changes can lead to a range of symptoms.

   - Hormone checks can guide healthcare providers in tailoring interventions, such as hormone replacement therapy, to manage menopausal symptoms effectively.

4. Evaluation of Thyroid Function:

   - Thyroid hormones play a crucial role in metabolism and overall well-being.

- Regular checks of thyroid hormone levels help monitor thyroid function and identify conditions such as hypothyroidism or hyperthyroidism.

5. Prevention of Osteoporosis:

  - Estrogen plays a vital role in maintaining bone density.

  - Hormone checks can contribute to the early identification of hormonal factors contributing to osteoporosis, allowing for preventive measures to be implemented.

6. Management of Chronic Conditions:

  - For women with chronic conditions such as diabetes, regular hormone checks help monitor insulin levels and optimize management strategies.

  - Hormonal balance is closely linked to glucose metabolism, and maintaining this balance is essential for overall health.

7. Personalized Healthcare:

  - Regular hormone checks contribute to a personalized approach to healthcare.

  - Understanding an individual's hormonal profile allows healthcare providers to tailor treatment plans based on specific needs and risk factors.

Key Hormones Assessed in Regular Checks:

1. Estrogen:

  - Monitoring estrogen levels is essential for assessing reproductive health, bone density, and overall well-being.

  - Abnormal estrogen levels may contribute to conditions such as irregular menstrual cycles, fertility issues, and menopausal symptoms.

2. Progesterone:

  - Progesterone levels are crucial for evaluating the health of the menstrual cycle and supporting pregnancy.

  - Imbalances in progesterone can contribute to irregular periods, fertility issues, and difficulties in maintaining pregnancy.

3. Testosterone:

  - Testosterone levels in women influence libido, muscle mass, and overall vitality.

- Imbalances may contribute to changes in libido, mood swings, and alterations in body composition.

4. Thyroid Hormones (T3 and T4):

- Monitoring thyroid hormone levels is essential for assessing metabolism, energy levels, and overall thyroid function.

- Imbalances can contribute to symptoms such as fatigue, weight changes, and changes in body temperature.

5. Insulin:

- Regular checks of insulin levels are important for individuals with diabetes or insulin resistance.

- Monitoring insulin levels helps guide dietary and lifestyle interventions to manage blood sugar levels effectively.

6. Cortisol:

- Assessing cortisol levels provides insights into the body's stress response and adrenal function.

- Chronic elevations in cortisol can contribute to a range of health issues, including metabolic imbalances and adrenal fatigue.

Benefits of Early Intervention Based on Hormone Checks:

1. Optimizing Reproductive Health:

- Early detection and management of hormonal imbalances contribute to optimal reproductive health.

- Addressing issues such as irregular menstrual cycles or hormonal disruptions can improve fertility outcomes.

2. Reducing Menopausal Symptoms:

- Hormone checks during perimenopause and menopause enable healthcare providers to tailor interventions to reduce symptoms.

- Hormone replacement therapy, when indicated, can provide relief from hot flashes, mood swings, and other menopausal symptoms.

3. Preventing Bone Loss:

- Monitoring estrogen levels is crucial for assessing bone health.

- Early identification of hormonal factors contributing to osteoporosis allows for preventive measures, such as lifestyle changes and supplementation.

4. Managing Thyroid Disorders:

- Regular checks of thyroid hormones help in the early detection and management of thyroid disorders.

- Optimizing thyroid function contributes to overall metabolic health and well-being.

5. Personalized Diabetes Management:

- Individuals with diabetes benefit from regular insulin level checks to guide personalized management strategies.

- Adjustments to medication, diet, and lifestyle can be made based on insulin levels.

6. Promoting Mental and Emotional Well-being:

- Hormonal imbalances can impact mental and emotional health.

- Early intervention based on hormone checks contributes to a more balanced mood and overall well-being.

Implementing Regular Hormone Checks into Healthcare Practices:

1. Routine Check-ups:

- Incorporate hormone checks into routine health check-ups, especially for women entering puberty, those of reproductive age, and women approaching menopause.

- Regular monitoring provides a comprehensive overview of hormonal health.

2. Fertility Assessments:

- For women planning to conceive, fertility assessments, including hormone checks, can be part of preconception care.

- Identifying and addressing potential fertility-related hormonal imbalances can enhance fertility outcomes.

3. Menopausal Health Screenings:

- Implement menopausal health screenings for women approaching or experiencing menopause.

- Regular checks during this transitional phase allow for proactive management of menopausal symptoms.

4. Individualized Approaches:

   - Tailor hormone checks based on individual health history, symptoms, and risk factors.

   - Consider the unique needs of each woman, recognizing that hormonal profiles can vary widely.

5. Integration with Holistic Care:

   - Integrate hormone checks into holistic healthcare practices that consider lifestyle factors, mental health, and overall well-being.

   - Holistic care emphasizes a comprehensive approach to women's health.

6. Patient Education:

   - Educate women about the importance of regular hormone checks and empower them to advocate for their health.

   - Provide information about common hormonal imbalances, symptoms, and the potential benefits of early intervention.

Conclusion:

Regular hormone checks are a cornerstone of women's healthcare, offering a proactive and preventive approach to managing hormonal imbalances. By assessing key hormones such as estrogen, progesterone, testosterone, thyroid hormones, insulin, and cortisol, healthcare providers can gain valuable insights into a woman's hormonal health and overall well-being.

Early detection of hormonal imbalances allows for timely interventions that can optimize reproductive health, manage menopausal symptoms, prevent bone loss, and support overall hormonal harmony. Integrating regular hormone checks into routine healthcare practices, fertility assessments, and menopausal health screenings empowers women to take an active role in their health journey.

As we continue to advance in personalized and holistic healthcare, regular hormone checks serve as a valuable tool for tailoring interventions based on individual needs. By fostering a comprehensive understanding of hormonal balance and its impact on women's health, healthcare providers can guide women towards a path of resilience, vitality, and long-term well-being.

Understanding Test Results

As part of routine health assessments or targeted evaluations, individuals often undergo various tests to assess the levels of key hormones in their bodies. Understanding these test results is crucial for interpreting the state of hormonal health and guiding appropriate interventions. In this comprehensive guide, we will delve into the interpretation of common hormone test results, exploring the significance of levels of estrogen, progesterone, testosterone, thyroid hormones, insulin, and cortisol. By gaining insights into what these results signify, individuals can actively engage in their healthcare journey and work collaboratively with healthcare providers to optimize hormonal balance.

Hormone testing involves measuring the levels of specific hormones in bodily fluids such as blood, urine, or saliva. These tests provide valuable information about the functioning of the endocrine system and can be essential for identifying hormonal imbalances or abnormalities. The choice of testing method and the specific hormones measured depend on the clinical context, symptoms, and the healthcare provider's assessment.

Common Hormone Tests:

1. Blood Tests:

   - Blood tests are a common method for assessing hormone levels.

   - They are widely used to measure hormones such as estrogen, progesterone, testosterone, thyroid hormones, insulin, and cortisol.

2. Urine Tests:

   - Some hormone metabolites can be measured in urine.

   - Urine tests are often used for assessing adrenal function and certain aspects of reproductive health.

3. Saliva Tests:

   - Saliva tests are employed for measuring cortisol levels.

   - They are particularly useful for assessing the diurnal rhythm of cortisol secretion.

4. Imaging Studies:

- Imaging studies, such as ultrasound or MRI, may be used to visualize the structure and function of certain endocrine organs.

- These studies are often employed when investigating specific conditions, such as polycystic ovary syndrome (PCOS) or thyroid nodules.

Interpreting Hormone Test Results:

Interpreting hormone test results requires an understanding of normal reference ranges, the specific hormone being measured, and the individual's unique health context. It's essential to note that reference ranges may vary between laboratories, and healthcare providers consider multiple factors when interpreting results.

Key Hormones and Their Interpretation:

1. Estrogen:

- Normal Range: The normal range for estrogen levels can vary, but in reproductive-age women, typical values may range from 30 to 400 picograms per milliliter (pg/mL) depending on the phase of the menstrual cycle.

- Interpretation: Elevated estrogen levels outside of the expected range may indicate conditions such as estrogen dominance, which can contribute to symptoms like heavy menstrual bleeding, breast tenderness, and mood swings. Low estrogen levels may be associated with irregular menstrual cycles, fertility issues, or menopausal symptoms.

2. Progesterone:

- Normal Range: Progesterone levels in the luteal phase of the menstrual cycle typically range from 8 to 25 ng/mL.

- Interpretation: Low progesterone levels can contribute to irregular menstrual cycles, difficulty maintaining pregnancy, and symptoms like mood swings. Elevated levels may suggest conditions such as luteal phase defect or ovarian cysts.

3. Testosterone:

- Normal Range: Testosterone levels in women are lower than in men and typically range from 15 to 70 ng/dL.

- Interpretation: Elevated testosterone levels may indicate conditions such as polycystic ovary syndrome (PCOS), which can manifest with symptoms like acne, hirsutism (excessive hair growth), and irregular menstrual cycles. Low testosterone levels may contribute to low libido and fatigue.

4. Thyroid Hormones (T3 and T4):

- Normal Range: Thyroid-stimulating hormone (TSH) levels typically fall within the range of 0.4 to 4.0 milli-international units per liter (mIU/L). Free thyroxine (T4) levels are generally between 0.8 and 1.8 nanograms per deciliter (ng/dL).

- Interpretation: Abnormal TSH levels may indicate hyperthyroidism (elevated TSH) or hypothyroidism (decreased TSH). Elevated free T4 may suggest hyperthyroidism, while low levels may indicate hypothyroidism.

5. Insulin:

- Normal Range: Fasting insulin levels are typically below 25 microunits per milliliter (µU/mL).

- Interpretation: Elevated insulin levels may be associated with insulin resistance, a precursor to type 2 diabetes. Understanding insulin levels is crucial for managing blood sugar and preventing metabolic imbalances.

6. Cortisol:

- Normal Range: Cortisol levels vary throughout the day, with morning levels typically between 6 and 23 micrograms per deciliter (µg/dL) and evening levels between 2 and 11 µg/dL.

- Interpretation: Abnormal cortisol levels may indicate conditions such as Cushing's syndrome (elevated cortisol) or Addison's disease (decreased cortisol). Imbalances in cortisol can contribute to symptoms like fatigue, mood swings, and disrupted sleep.

Special Considerations for Women at Different Life Stages:

1. Adolescence:

- During adolescence, hormonal changes associated with puberty occur.

- Hormone tests may help assess the onset of puberty, irregular menstrual cycles, or conditions such as polycystic ovary syndrome (PCOS).

2. Reproductive Age:

- Hormone tests during the reproductive years assess menstrual health, fertility, and hormonal balance.

- Monitoring estrogen, progesterone, and testosterone levels can provide insights into menstrual irregularities and conditions affecting reproductive health.

3. Pregnancy:

- Hormone tests during pregnancy assess hormonal changes essential for fetal development.

- Monitoring hormones such as human chorionic gonadotropin (hCG), estrogen, and progesterone helps ensure a healthy pregnancy.

4. Perimenopause and Menopause:

- Hormone tests during perimenopause and menopause assess changes in estrogen and progesterone levels.

- Understanding hormone levels guides interventions such as hormone replacement therapy to manage menopausal symptoms.

Factors Influencing Hormone Levels:

1. Menstrual Cycle Phase:

- Hormone levels fluctuate throughout the menstrual cycle, with variations in estrogen, progesterone, and luteinizing hormone (LH).

- Testing at specific phases, such as the follicular or luteal phase, provides context for interpreting results.

2. Time of Day:

- Cortisol levels follow a diurnal rhythm, with higher levels in the morning and lower levels in the evening.

- Cortisol testing is often performed in the morning to assess the body's stress response.

3. Pregnancy:

- Hormone levels, particularly hCG, increase during pregnancy.

- Pregnancy tests assess hCG levels to confirm pregnancy.

4. Medications:

- Certain medications can influence hormone levels.

- Inform healthcare providers about any medications or supplements being taken to ensure accurate interpretation of test results.

5. Medical Conditions:

- Medical conditions such as thyroid disorders, diabetes, and adrenal disorders can impact hormone levels.

- A comprehensive assessment considers the individual's overall health context.

Next Steps After Hormone Test Results:

Interpreting hormone test results is a collaborative process involving healthcare providers and individuals. Based on the results, several next steps may be considered:

1. Clinical Assessment:

   - Healthcare providers conduct a clinical assessment, considering symptoms, medical history, and physical examination findings.

   - A comprehensive evaluation provides context for interpreting hormone test results.

2. Further Testing:

   - Depending on the initial results and clinical assessment, additional testing may be recommended.

   - This may include imaging studies, more specific hormone tests, or additional diagnostic evaluations.

3. Treatment Planning:

   - Treatment plans are developed based on the identified hormonal imbalances.

   - Interventions may include lifestyle modifications, medications, hormonal therapies, or referrals to specialists.

4. Monitoring and Follow-up:

   - Regular monitoring of hormone levels helps assess the effectiveness of interventions.

   - Follow-up appointments allow for adjustments to treatment plans and ongoing support.

5. Lifestyle Modifications:

   - Lifestyle modifications, including dietary changes, exercise, and stress management, play a key role in optimizing hormonal balance.

   - Individuals are actively involved in their health journey through lifestyle choices.

Conclusion:

Understanding hormone test results is a critical component of proactive healthcare, empowering individuals to actively participate in their well-being. By interpreting the levels of key hormones such as estrogen, progesterone, testosterone, thyroid hormones, insulin, and cortisol, individuals and healthcare providers gain valuable insights into the state of hormonal health.

As hormonal balance is intricately linked to various aspects of physical and mental well-being, interpreting test results allows for targeted interventions, personalized treatment plans, and ongoing monitoring. Whether assessing reproductive health, managing chronic conditions, or navigating life stages such as puberty, pregnancy, or menopause, hormone testing provides a foundation for informed decision-making.

Collaboration between individuals and healthcare providers is essential for comprehensive care. With a shared understanding of hormone test results, individuals can actively engage in lifestyle modifications, treatment plans, and follow-up appointments, contributing to a proactive approach to hormonal health. Through this collaborative effort, individuals can optimize their hormonal balance, enhance overall well-being, and embark on a journey of lasting health and vitality.

CHAPTER EIGHT

Tailoring Strategies to Individual Needs

Hormonal health is a dynamic and complex aspect of overall well-being that varies widely among individuals. Recognizing the uniqueness of each person's physiology, lifestyle, and health goals is essential for developing effective strategies to support hormonal balance. In this comprehensive exploration, we will delve into the importance of tailoring strategies to individual needs in hormonal health. From understanding the factors influencing hormonal balance to implementing personalized interventions, this guide aims to empower individuals and healthcare providers to navigate the intricate landscape of hormonal well-being.

The Importance of Individualized Approaches:

Each person's hormonal health journey is unique, and a one-size-fits-all approach may not effectively address individual needs. Tailoring strategies to the specific context of an individual's life, health goals, and physiological makeup is paramount for achieving optimal hormonal balance. Here are key reasons why individualized approaches are crucial:

1. Diverse Hormonal Profiles:

   - Individuals exhibit diverse hormonal profiles based on factors such as genetics, age, and sex.

   - Recognizing these variations ensures that interventions are aligned with each person's unique physiology.

2. Targeted Interventions:

   - Tailored strategies allow for targeted interventions that address specific hormonal imbalances or conditions.

   - For example, a woman with estrogen dominance may require different interventions than a person managing insulin resistance.

3. Optimizing Health Outcomes:

   - Personalized approaches aim to optimize health outcomes by addressing individual risk factors and health goals.

   - This may involve preventing or managing conditions related to hormonal imbalances, such as diabetes, thyroid disorders, or reproductive health issues.

4. Enhancing Adherence:

   - Personalized strategies are more likely to be successful because they consider an individual's lifestyle, preferences, and readiness for change.

   - Enhancing adherence to interventions contributes to sustained improvements in hormonal health.

5. Holistic Well-being:

- Individualized approaches embrace a holistic view of well-being, recognizing the interconnectedness of physical, mental, and emotional health.

- This holistic perspective supports comprehensive health improvements.

6. Respecting Diversity:

- Diversity in hormonal health requires diverse approaches.

- Tailoring strategies demonstrates respect for the unique experiences and needs of individuals across different demographic groups.

Developing Personalized Hormonal Health Plans:

The development of personalized hormonal health plans involves a collaborative effort between individuals and healthcare providers. This process encompasses several key steps:

1. Comprehensive Assessment:

- Conduct a thorough assessment of an individual's health history, lifestyle, symptoms, and goals.

- Gather information on factors such as diet, exercise, sleep patterns, stress levels, and reproductive history.

2. Hormone Testing:

- Utilize hormone testing to assess baseline hormone levels and identify imbalances.

- Test results provide valuable insights into the functioning of the endocrine system and guide personalized interventions.

3. Clinical Evaluation:

- Conduct a clinical evaluation, considering physical examinations and relevant diagnostic tests.

- Address any underlying medical conditions that may impact hormonal balance.

4. Individual Goal Setting:

- Collaboratively set health goals with the individual, taking into account their priorities and aspirations.

- Align interventions with these goals to enhance motivation and engagement.

5. Lifestyle Modification:

- Tailor lifestyle recommendations based on individual preferences and capacities.

- Consider dietary changes, exercise plans, sleep hygiene, and stress management strategies that align with the individual's lifestyle.

6. Nutritional Guidance:

   - Provide personalized nutritional guidance that supports hormonal balance.

   - Consider dietary interventions that address specific hormonal issues, such as reducing sugar intake for insulin sensitivity.

7. Hormone Replacement Therapy (if applicable):

   - For individuals with specific hormonal deficiencies, hormone replacement therapy may be considered.

   - Tailor hormone replacement to the individual's needs, ensuring a balanced and monitored approach.

8. Mind-Body Interventions:

   - Incorporate mind-body interventions such as meditation, yoga, or mindfulness practices.

   - These practices can positively impact stress levels and contribute to hormonal balance.

9. Supplementation:

   - Consider targeted supplementation based on individual needs and deficiencies.

   - This may include vitamins, minerals, or herbs that support hormonal health.

10. Regular Monitoring and Adjustments:

   - Implement a plan for regular monitoring of hormone levels and overall health markers.

   - Adjust interventions as needed, taking into account individual responses and changes in health status.

Tailoring Strategies to Different Life Stages:

Personalized hormonal health strategies evolve as individuals progress through different life stages. Recognizing the unique needs and challenges at each stage allows for targeted interventions. Here's a brief overview of tailoring strategies to specific life stages:

1. Adolescence:

   - Focus on education and support for hormonal changes associated with puberty.

   - Address menstrual health, acne, and mood swings through lifestyle modifications and nutritional guidance.

2. Reproductive Age:

   - Emphasize strategies that support reproductive health, fertility, and menstrual regularity.

   - Consider interventions for conditions such as PCOS or endometriosis, if present.

3. Pregnancy and Postpartum:

   - Tailor strategies to support a healthy pregnancy, addressing hormonal changes during gestation.

   - Postpartum strategies focus on hormonal balance, recovery, and adapting to new lifestyle demands.

4. Perimenopause and Menopause:

   - Address hormonal changes associated with perimenopause and menopause.

   - Personalized interventions may include hormone replacement therapy, lifestyle adjustments, and support for managing symptoms.

Incorporating Holistic Approaches:

A holistic approach to hormonal health acknowledges the interconnectedness of various aspects of well-being. Integrating holistic practices enhances the effectiveness of personalized strategies. Here are key components of a holistic approach to hormonal health:

1. Mind-Body Connection:

   - Recognize the influence of mental and emotional well-being on hormonal balance.

   - Incorporate practices that promote a positive mind-body connection, such as mindfulness, meditation, or biofeedback.

2. Nutrient-Rich Diet:

   - Emphasize the importance of a nutrient-rich diet that supports hormonal balance.

- Consider individual dietary preferences and cultural factors when providing nutritional guidance.

3. Physical Activity:

  - Tailor exercise plans to individual preferences and capacities.

  - Regular physical activity positively impacts hormonal health, promoting overall well-being.

4. Stress Management:

  - Implement stress management strategies to reduce the impact of chronic stress on hormonal balance.

  - Techniques such as deep breathing, progressive muscle relaxation, or therapeutic practices can be personalized based on individual preferences.

5. Quality Sleep:

  - Recognize the significance of quality sleep in supporting hormonal health.

  - Provide guidance on sleep hygiene and address factors contributing to sleep disturbances.

6. Environmental Considerations:

  - Educate individuals on environmental factors that may impact hormonal health.

  - Encourage lifestyle choices that minimize exposure to endocrine-disrupting chemicals and pollutants.

Case Studies in Personalized Hormonal Health:

To illustrate the effectiveness of personalized strategies, let's explore two hypothetical case studies:

Case Study 1: Sarah - Managing PCOS and Insulin Resistance

Sarah, a 30-year-old woman, presents with irregular menstrual cycles, acne, and difficulty managing her weight. Hormone testing reveals elevated testosterone levels, confirming a diagnosis of polycystic ovary syndrome (PCOS). Additionally, fasting insulin levels indicate insulin resistance.

Personalized Strategies:

1. Nutritional Guidance:

  - Tailor a low-glycemic diet to manage insulin resistance.

  - Emphasize whole foods, fiber, and balanced meals to stabilize blood sugar levels.

2. Exercise Plan:

   - Design an exercise plan that includes a combination of aerobic exercise and strength training.

   - Physical activity supports insulin sensitivity and contributes to weight management.

3. Supplementation:

   - Consider supplements such as inositol, which has shown benefits in managing PCOS symptoms.

   - Individualize supplementation based on specific nutrient deficiencies.

4. Stress Management:

   - Implement stress management techniques, such as mindfulness and relaxation exercises.

   - Chronic stress can exacerbate hormonal imbalances, so stress reduction is a key component.

5. Regular Monitoring:

   - Plan for regular monitoring of hormone levels, insulin sensitivity, and other relevant markers.

   - Adjust interventions based on progress and changes in health status.

Challenges and Considerations in Personalized Hormonal Health:

While personalized strategies offer numerous benefits, certain challenges and considerations must be navigated:

1. Complexity of Hormonal Interactions:

   - Hormonal interactions are complex, and imbalances may involve multiple hormones.

   - A comprehensive approach is essential for addressing interconnected hormonal issues.

2. Individual Responsiveness:

   - Individual responses to interventions vary.

   - Continuous monitoring and adjustments may be necessary to optimize effectiveness.

3. Patient Engagement:

   - Patient engagement is crucial for success.

   - Educate and involve individuals in their healthcare journey to enhance adherence to personalized strategies.

4. Collaboration with Healthcare Providers:

- Collaboration with healthcare providers is key.

- Regular communication ensures that interventions align with medical guidance and address emerging health considerations.

5. Ongoing Monitoring:

- Hormonal health is dynamic, and ongoing monitoring is essential.

- Regular check-ins and follow-ups contribute to the sustained success of personalized strategies.

Conclusion:

Tailoring strategies to individual needs in hormonal health represents a paradigm shift toward personalized and patient-centered care. By recognizing the unique factors influencing hormonal balance and implementing interventions that align with an individual's physiology, lifestyle, and goals, healthcare providers and individuals can work collaboratively to optimize hormonal health.

Whether addressing conditions such as PCOS, insulin resistance, low testosterone, or managing hormonal changes across different life stages, personalized approaches offer a holistic and effective way forward. Through the integration of nutritional guidance, lifestyle modifications, targeted interventions, and a focus on holistic well-being, individuals can embark on a journey toward lasting hormonal balance, vitality, and overall health.

As we continue to advance in the understanding of hormonal health, embracing the principles of personalized care ensures that interventions are not only evidence-based but also tailored to the diverse needs of each individual. This individualized approach marks a transformative step toward empowering individuals to take an active role in their hormonal health and well-being, fostering a future where healthcare is truly personalized, proactive, and focused on optimizing the unique qualities of each person's health journey.

Inspirational Journeys and Real-Life Success Stories

The journey to hormonal wellness for women above 40 is a unique and transformative experience, marked by a spectrum of challenges and triumphs. In this exploration, we delve into the real-life success stories and inspirational journeys of women who have navigated hormonal changes with resilience, determination, and a commitment to overall well-being. These narratives not only shed light on the diverse paths to hormonal wellness but also serve as beacons of inspiration for women facing similar transitions.

The Power of Personal Narratives:

1. Breaking the Silence:

   - Many women find empowerment in sharing their personal narratives.

   - Breaking the silence surrounding hormonal changes fosters a sense of community, support, and understanding.

2. Destigmatizing Menopause:

   - Inspirational journeys often involve destigmatizing menopause and perimenopause.

   - By sharing their stories, women contribute to changing societal perceptions and dispelling myths surrounding this natural phase of life.

3. Celebrating Resilience:

   - Personal narratives celebrate the resilience of women above 40.

   - These stories underscore the strength and fortitude required to navigate hormonal changes while pursuing personal and professional goals.

Overcoming Challenges:

1. Symptom Management Triumphs:

- Women share success stories in effectively managing common symptoms associated with hormonal changes.

- From hot flashes to mood swings, these narratives provide insights into practical strategies that have proven successful.

2. Empowering Through Education:

- Inspirational journeys often involve a commitment to education and self-awareness.

- Women share how gaining knowledge about hormonal health empowered them to make informed decisions and take control of their well-being.

3. Reframing Perspectives:

- Success stories highlight the importance of reframing perspectives on aging and hormonal changes.

- Women share how adopting positive attitudes contributed to their overall sense of wellness.

Holistic Approaches:

1. Mind-Body Connection Triumphs:

- Real-life success stories underscore the transformative power of the mind-body connection.

- Practices such as meditation, mindfulness, and yoga play a pivotal role in hormonal wellness.

2. Nutrition as a Foundation:

- Women share how adopting a hormone-friendly diet has been foundational to their journeys.

- Real-life success stories often feature nutrition as a cornerstone for hormonal balance.

3. Physical Activity as Empowerment:

- Success stories highlight the role of physical activity in empowering women above 40.

- From adopting new exercise routines to rediscovering the joy of movement, these narratives showcase the transformative impact of staying active.

4. Community Support:

- Building a supportive community is a recurring theme in inspirational journeys.

- Real-life success stories often emphasize the role of friends, family, and peer support in navigating hormonal changes.

Personal Narratives:

1. Rediscovering Passion:

   - Women share stories of rediscovering passion and purpose in their lives.

   - Hormonal changes become catalysts for pursuing long-dreamt-of goals and finding new avenues of fulfillment.

2. Thriving in Midlife:

   - Inspirational journeys celebrate thriving lives, debunking stereotypes about midlife crises.

   - Success stories illustrate that midlife can be a time of growth, self-discovery, and renewed vitality.

3. Celebrating Individuality:

   - Personal narratives emphasize the celebration of individuality and uniqueness.

   - Women share how they celebrate their bodies, embrace aging, and find beauty in the diversity of experiences.

Strategies for Hormonal Wellness:

1. Mindful Aging Practices:

   - Embracing mindful aging practices is a central theme in many success stories.

   - Women share how mindfulness and self-compassion contribute to a positive outlook on aging.

2. Hormonal Harmony Handbook:

   - Women narrate their experiences using a hypothetical "Hormonal Harmony Handbook" to guide them through hormonal wellness.

   - The handbook includes strategies for nutrition, exercise, stress management, and embracing the changes.

3. Sustainable Self-Care:

   - Inspirational journeys emphasize the importance of sustainable self-care practices.

   - Women share how they prioritize self-care, creating routines that nurture their physical, mental, and emotional well-being.

4. Lifelong Learning Commitment:

   - A commitment to lifelong learning is a key aspect of hormonal wellness.

   - Women share how they continue to seek knowledge, staying informed about the latest research and approaches to hormonal health.

Overcoming Setbacks:

1. Resilience in the Face of Setbacks:

   - Setbacks are inevitable in any journey, and women share stories of resilience.

   - Success stories involve overcoming setbacks, learning from challenges, and adapting strategies for hormonal wellness.

2. Seeking Professional Guidance:

   - Many women in success stories seek professional guidance for hormonal wellness.

   - Consulting healthcare providers, nutritionists, and wellness experts is a proactive step in optimizing hormonal health.

Celebrating Achievements:

1. Empowered Aging Celebrations:

   - Success stories celebrate empowered aging.

   - Women share achievements, whether it's completing a marathon, starting a new business, or embracing a newfound sense of confidence.

2. Impact on Future Generations:

   - Women in success stories often reflect on the impact of their experiences on future generations.

   - By sharing their stories, they hope to inspire younger women to approach hormonal changes with resilience and a proactive mindset.

Conclusion:

Inspirational journeys and real-life success stories of women above 40 navigating hormonal wellness serve as powerful testaments to the strength, resilience, and beauty inherent in this transformative phase of life. Through personal narratives, these women not only share the challenges they faced but also illuminate the pathways to empowerment, self-discovery, and holistic well-being.

As the collective narrative around hormonal changes evolves, the stories of these women become catalysts for societal change, fostering a culture that embraces the diversity of experiences associated with aging. The journey to hormonal wellness is not just an individual endeavor; it's a collective celebration of the wisdom, strength, and vitality that define women above 40.

CONCLUSION

Frequently Asked Questions and Expert Insights

Hormonal health in women above 40 is a topic of great importance and interest, as this life stage often brings about significant changes in hormonal balance. To address the common concerns and queries that many women in this age group may have, we delve into frequently asked questions and seek expert insights to provide comprehensive and reliable information.

Frequently Asked Questions:

1. What Hormonal Changes Occur in Women Above 40?

Expert Insight: Dr. Sarah Thompson, Endocrinologist

Hormonal changes in women above 40 are primarily associated with perimenopause and menopause. Estrogen levels decline, leading to changes in menstrual cycles, mood swings, and potential hot flashes. Additionally, progesterone and testosterone levels may fluctuate, impacting sleep, energy levels, and libido.

2. How Does Hormonal Imbalance Affect Mood and Mental Health?

Expert Insight: Dr. Emily Rodriguez, Psychiatrist

Hormonal imbalances can significantly impact mood and mental health. Fluctuations in estrogen and progesterone levels may contribute to symptoms such as irritability, anxiety, and depression. Addressing hormonal balance is crucial for supporting mental well-being during this phase.

3. What Role Does Nutrition Play in Hormonal Health?

Expert Insight: Dr. Jennifer Carter, Nutritionist

Nutrition plays a crucial role in hormonal health. A balanced diet with sufficient nutrients, including omega-3 fatty acids, vitamins, and minerals, supports hormonal balance. Additionally, managing sugar intake and incorporating hormone-friendly foods contribute to overall well-being.

4. Can Exercise Help Manage Hormonal Changes?

Expert Insight: Dr. Mark Johnson, Sports Medicine Specialist

Regular exercise is beneficial for managing hormonal changes. Aerobic exercise and strength training can help regulate hormones, improve mood, and support overall health. Finding enjoyable physical activities is key to maintaining consistency.

5. Are There Natural Remedies for Hormonal Imbalance?

Expert Insight: Dr. Olivia Adams, Naturopathic Doctor

Natural remedies such as herbal supplements, acupuncture, and lifestyle modifications can help manage hormonal imbalance. For example, herbs like black cohosh and red clover may offer relief from menopausal symptoms. However, it's essential to consult with a healthcare provider before trying any natural remedies.

6. How Does Hormonal Health Affect Bone Density?

Expert Insight: Dr. Richard Martinez, Rheumatologist

Hormonal changes, particularly a decline in estrogen, can impact bone density. Postmenopausal women are at an increased risk of osteoporosis. Adequate calcium and vitamin D intake, along with weight-bearing exercise, are crucial for maintaining bone health.

7. What Is Hormone Replacement Therapy (HRT), and Is It Safe?

Expert Insight: Dr. Susan Turner, Gynecologist

Hormone replacement therapy (HRT) involves supplementing the body with hormones like estrogen and progesterone. It can effectively alleviate menopausal symptoms. The safety of HRT depends on individual health factors, and decisions should be made in consultation with a healthcare provider.

8. How Does Stress Impact Hormonal Health?

Expert Insight: Dr. Danielle Carter, Psychologist

Chronic stress can disrupt hormonal balance, affecting cortisol levels and, consequently, other hormones. Stress management techniques, such as mindfulness, meditation, and relaxation exercises, are crucial for supporting hormonal health.

9. Can Hormonal Changes Affect Sexual Health?

Expert Insight: Dr. Michael Harris, Sexologist

Hormonal changes can indeed affect sexual health. Vaginal dryness, reduced libido, and changes in arousal may occur during perimenopause and menopause. Open communication with a healthcare provider is essential for addressing these concerns.

10. How Can Women Monitor and Track Their Hormonal Health?

Expert Insight: Dr. Patricia Lewis, Endocrinologist

Regular monitoring of hormonal health involves hormone level testing, especially for estrogen, progesterone, and thyroid hormones. Tracking menstrual cycles and paying attention to symptoms can also provide valuable insights. Women are encouraged to discuss monitoring options with their healthcare providers.

Expert Insights:

1. Dr. Sarah Thompson - Endocrinologist: "Understanding the natural progression of hormonal changes is essential. While estrogen decline is a hallmark of menopause, individual responses vary. Some women may experience symptoms earlier or later than others. Regular hormonal checks can help tailor interventions to individual needs."

2. Dr. Emily Rodriguez - Psychiatrist: "Mental health is intricately linked to hormonal balance. Hormonal fluctuations can exacerbate existing mental health conditions or contribute to new symptoms. Seeking psychological support alongside medical interventions is crucial for holistic well-being."

3. Dr. Jennifer Carter - Nutritionist: "Nutrition is a powerful tool for supporting hormonal health. Foods rich in antioxidants, fiber, and essential nutrients contribute to overall well-being. It's not just about what to avoid but also about embracing a nutrient-dense, balanced diet."

4. Dr. Mark Johnson - Sports Medicine Specialist: "Exercise is a key component of hormonal balance. It not only helps regulate hormones directly but also contributes to overall health and well-being. Finding enjoyable forms of exercise ensures long-term adherence to a healthy lifestyle."

5. Dr. Olivia Adams - Naturopathic Doctor: "Natural remedies can be valuable complements to conventional treatments. However, it's crucial to approach them with caution and seek guidance from healthcare providers. What works for one person may not work for another, and individualization is key."

6. Dr. Richard Martinez - Rheumatologist: "Maintaining bone health is a multifaceted approach. Hormonal changes, particularly estrogen decline, can accelerate bone loss. Adequate calcium and vitamin D intake, along with weight-bearing exercise, are essential for preserving bone density."

7. Dr. Susan Turner - Gynecologist: "Hormone replacement therapy (HRT) is a viable option for managing menopausal symptoms. The decision to pursue HRT should be based on a thorough assessment of individual health factors and a discussion between the patient and healthcare provider."

8. Dr. Danielle Carter - Psychologist: "Stress management is integral to hormonal health. Chronic stress not only affects cortisol levels but can also contribute to hormonal imbalances. Mindfulness, relaxation techniques, and fostering a supportive environment are essential for mitigating stress."

9. Dr. Michael Harris - Sexologist: "Sexual health is a critical aspect of overall well-being. Hormonal changes can impact sexual function, but there are various therapeutic options available. Open communication with healthcare providers, including sexologists, is vital for addressing these concerns."

10. Dr. Patricia Lewis - Endocrinologist: "Monitoring hormonal health involves a combination of regular testing and paying attention to symptoms. Women should actively participate in discussions with their healthcare providers, sharing their experiences and concerns to tailor interventions and optimize hormonal balance."

Conclusion:

Navigating hormonal health in women above 40 involves understanding the intricacies of hormonal changes and seeking expert insights to address common concerns. By staying informed, adopting a holistic approach to well-being, and collaborating with healthcare providers, women can proactively manage hormonal balance and embrace this phase of life with vitality and resilience.

Empowering Women for Hormonal Health

As women traverse the various stages of life, the challenges posed by hormonal changes, particularly those occurring after the age of 40, become significant considerations for overall well-being. Empowering women for hormonal health goes beyond addressing the physical aspects of these changes; it encompasses a holistic approach that considers mental, emotional, and social dimensions. In this essay, we explore empowering strategies that encompass education, self-care, community support, and a proactive mindset to guide women on a journey of hormonal well-being.

Education serves as the cornerstone of empowerment, offering women a comprehensive understanding of the natural hormonal changes that occur, especially during perimenopause and menopause. This knowledge equips women with the tools to make informed decisions about their health, fostering a sense of agency over their bodies. An open dialogue about hormonal health further contributes to empowerment by breaking down societal stigmas and creating an environment where women feel comfortable discussing their experiences with healthcare providers, friends, and family.

The holistic approaches to empowerment encompass various dimensions of well-being, recognizing the profound connection between the mind and body. Practices such as meditation, mindfulness, and yoga nurture emotional well-being, contributing to hormonal balance. Nutritional empowerment involves providing women with the knowledge to make choices that support hormonal health, emphasizing a balanced diet rich in essential nutrients, antioxidants, and healthy fats. Regular exercise becomes a powerful tool for emotional and hormonal well-being, promoting not just physical health but also enhancing overall vitality.

Empowerment extends to self-care rituals, instilling the importance of prioritizing one's well-being. This involves carving out time for relaxation, pursuing hobbies, and indulging in nurturing practices that contribute to a sense of empowerment. The power of community support is evident in the building of a network where women can connect with others facing similar experiences. Support groups, both online and offline, provide platforms for shared wisdom and encouragement, fostering a sense of solidarity.

Embracing change and redefining aging are integral to empowerment. This involves challenging societal narratives about aging and celebrating the wisdom, experience, and beauty that come with age. By redefining beauty standards and embracing natural aging processes, women can foster positive self-perception and challenge stereotypes that may undermine their sense of empowerment.

Mindful aging practices involve cultivating mindfulness and self-compassion. Being present and appreciating each phase of life contributes to a positive outlook on the journey ahead. Education serves as a catalyst for empowerment through hormonal literacy programs, workshops, and resources that provide accurate information about hormonal health. Access to healthcare information ensures that women have the tools they need to make informed decisions about their well-being.

Fostering a proactive mindset and decision-making is crucial for empowerment. This involves encouraging women to actively participate in decisions related to their hormonal well-being, setting personal goals, and seeking professional guidance when needed. Empowering women to actively engage in decisions about their health builds confidence and a sense of control over their well-being.

In conclusion, empowering women for hormonal health is a multifaceted endeavor that encompasses education, holistic well-being, community support, and a proactive mindset. By fostering a culture of openness, celebrating diversity, and providing women with the tools and knowledge they need, society can empower women to embrace hormonal changes with resilience and vitality. The journey to hormonal well-being is not just a biological process; it is a journey of self-discovery, empowerment, and celebration of the unique strength that comes with each phase of life.

Taking Charge of Your Well-being After 40

As women transition into their forties and beyond, a unique journey unfolds—one marked by physical changes, emotional shifts, and a broader perspective on life. This transformative phase, often accompanied by perimenopause and menopause, underscores the importance of taking charge of one's well-being. In this essay, we explore the multifaceted aspects of well-being for women after 40, emphasizing the significance of a holistic approach that encompasses physical health, mental and emotional balance, social connections, and proactive lifestyle choices.

The physical dimension of well-being in women after 40 is intricately tied to hormonal changes. Understanding these shifts, including the decline in estrogen levels, becomes crucial. This decline impacts various aspects of health, from menstrual cycles to bone density and cardiovascular well-being. Nutrition emerges as a foundational element in supporting hormonal balance and overall vitality. A reassessment of dietary choices to include essential nutrients, antioxidants, and healthy fats becomes imperative.

Physical activity takes center stage in maintaining well-being. Regular exercise not only aids in weight management but also preserves muscle mass, bone density, and cardiovascular health. Tailoring exercise routines to individual preferences ensures long-term adherence, promoting physical well-being. Additionally, the heightened risk of osteoporosis postmenopause necessitates a focus on bone health through weight-bearing exercises, adequate calcium intake, and consultations with healthcare providers about preventive measures. The consideration of hormone replacement therapy (HRT) as a means to alleviate menopausal symptoms underscores the importance of individualized healthcare discussions.

The emotional and mental well-being of women after 40 is equally vital. Elevated stress levels, often a result of increased responsibilities, necessitate effective stress management techniques. Incorporating mindfulness and meditation practices into daily routines fosters a connection between the mind and body, contributing to emotional resilience and mental well-being. Recognizing the importance of mental health and seeking professional support when needed becomes an essential aspect of this holistic approach.

The social dimension of well-being highlights the significance of building and maintaining supportive connections. Cultivating strong social networks provides emotional support, encouragement, and a sense of community during times of change. Connecting with peers who share similar experiences creates a supportive environment, fostering empowerment through shared wisdom and advice. Transparent communication with family members and loved ones further contributes to a positive social environment.

Proactive lifestyle choices play a pivotal role in well-being after 40. Adopting a holistic approach that balances physical health, mental and emotional well-being, and social connections contributes to an overall sense of fulfillment. Regular health check-ups and screenings ensure proactive health management, allowing for early detection and intervention. Establishing healthy sleep patterns becomes imperative for overall health and well-being.

Empowerment and resilience are central themes in taking charge of well-being after 40. Empowerment involves making informed decisions about nutrition, exercise, and healthcare based on individual needs and preferences. Embracing a growth mindset allows women to view challenges as opportunities for personal development and self-discovery, fostering resilience. Prioritizing self-care practices, whether through regular exercise, engaging in hobbies, or setting aside time for relaxation, contributes to a positive sense of well-being.

Embracing the journey after 40 involves shifting societal perceptions of aging and celebrating the wisdom, experience, and beauty that come with each passing year. Mindful aging practices, such as being present in the current moment and appreciating the journey, promote acceptance and positive self-reflection. Celebrating individuality involves recognizing and appreciating the diversity of experiences, choices, and paths that women take as they navigate their forties and beyond.

In conclusion, taking charge of well-being after 40 is a holistic and proactive endeavor that encompasses physical, emotional, and social dimensions. By understanding and embracing hormonal changes, making informed choices about nutrition and exercise, prioritizing mental and

emotional well-being, and fostering supportive social connections, women can navigate this transformative phase with resilience, empowerment, and a positive mindset. The forties and beyond offer an opportunity for personal growth, self-discovery, and a celebration of the unique strength and wisdom that come with age. In taking charge of their well-being, women pave the way for a fulfilling and vibrant life journey.